The List

Judith Tydor Baumel-Schwartz (ed.)

The List

The Making of an Online Transnational Second Generation Community

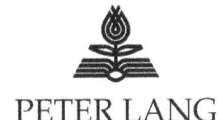

PETER LANG

Bern · Berlin · Bruxelles · New York · Oxford

Bibliographic Information published by the Deutsche Nationalbibliothek
The Deutsche Nationalbibliothek lists this publication in the Deutsche Nationalbibliografie; detailed bibliographic data is available online at http://dnb.d-nb.de.

Library of Congress Cataloging-in-Publication Data
A CIP catalog record for this book has been applied for at the Library of Congress

This book is published with the generous assistance of the Finkler Institute of Holocaust Research and the Koschitsky Fund of the Israel and Golda Koschtisky Department of Jewish History and Contemporary Jewry at Bar-Ilan University, Ramat Gan, Israel

ISBN 978-3-0343-4439-5 (Print)
E-ISBN 978-3-0343-4470-8 (E-PDF)
E-ISBN 978-3-0343-4471-5 (EPUB)
DOI 10.3726/b19323

© Peter Lang Group AG, International Academic Publishers, Bern 2022
Bern@peterlang.com, www.peterlang.com

All rights reserved.
This publication has been peer reviewed.

All parts of this publication are protected by copyright. Any utilisation outside the strict limits of the copyright law, without the permission of the publisher, is forbidden and liable to prosecution. This applies in particular to reproductions, translations, microfilming, and storage and processing in electronic retrieval systems.

Dedicated to our children and grandchildren, the 3rd and 4th Generations, in the hope that it will help them understand us better

Table of Contents

Dr. Eva Fogelman
Preface: Generations of the Holocaust: Invisible to Visible
Identity and Community 9

Prof. Judith Tydor Baumel-Schwartz
Introduction 27

Marilyn Boehm
From the Ashes to a Flame 37

Dr. Paula David
The Outsider on the Inside 53

Patrice Flesch
The Lie 69

Paul Foldes
The List Creator's Story 81

Martin Herskovitz
How The List Transformed My Life 93

Clara Jacob
You've Got 2G Mail 113

Gail Ellen Rubinstein Lipton
My Journey – Discovery, Connection, and Community 129

Dr. Betty Unger Needleman
My 2G Life and My Virtual Community 141

Prof. Judith Tydor Baumel-Schwartz
My Life in Lists 153

Jeanette Friedman Sieradski
Taaseh Lach Chavurah **– Create Your Own 'Hood** 169

Laurie Solnik
You Can't Know What You Don't Know 183

Dr. Ruth Samuel Tenenholtz
We Are Family: A Journey With the 2G Discussion List 199

Notes on Contributors 213

Dr. Eva Fogelman
Preface: Generations of the Holocaust: Invisible to Visible Identity and Community

Introduction

I was born in a half-burned-out hospital in Kassel, Germany. Ninety percent of its old city was bombed to smithereens by the Allies during World War II. The medieval buildings and the city center were devastated during a seven-day fire, which killed 10,000 Germans, and quarter of a million people were homeless, including my parents. They were two Holocaust survivors who met soon after the war, by chance, on a bus not far from Munich. My mother, Leah Burstyn, was traveling with her brother, George.

My father, Simcha Fagelman, approached them and asked if they knew of a place where he and his comrade could live. My mother suggested they all go together to the Goldkopf Displaced Persons Camp, where the four new friends started a business of buying and selling cigarettes, chocolates, and other goods.

There were rumors saying that pregnant women and elderly Jews could be transferred to row houses in a Displaced Persons Camp in Kassel, so my mother put a pillow over her stomach, covered it with a coat, and before they were married, stood in line with my father to role play a pregnant woman. It worked. They got an attached row house.

My Family

My mother was the youngest of five children in the Burstyn family and grew up in Wyshkow, a town on the Bug River, 55 km northeast of Warsaw on the highway to Bialystok. Of the 12,650 residents, 45 % were Jews of all persuasions, from HaShomer HaTzair Zionists to Hasidim. When the Germans invaded the area, the Jews were the most vulnerable. At the start, 65 Jews were killed. Houses with Friday night candles were set on fire. The synagogues, *shtibelach* (usually a room in a rabbi's family home that served as a small synagogue), and the Beit Midrash (House of Study) were burned to the ground. My mother's family managed, with a few meager possessions, to get a ride on a horse and buggy. The most important items they took were blankets and pillows. Bombs dropped around them, left and right, but they managed to dodge them. Others were fleeing east as well, and they were not that lucky. The family rode from one town to another without food and slept along the way. A week later they arrived in Stocheck-Wengrofsky and stayed for three months. The Burstyn clan then continued towards the Bug River and arranged to cross it. Eventually they got to Bialystok and went to the first place they could think of – the synagogue. It was packed with people, so that night, the family slept on the street. Luckily, a relative got them an apartment where they were able to stay for a few months.

The German troops, following the same route, soon reached Bialystok, and the Burstyns again fled the bombs, heading east to Orsha, near Minsk, Belarus, where they were incarcerated in a slave labor camp for 18 months, from April 1940 until October 1941. After being released, they continued heading east by train, almost starved to death, and eventually came to Tashkent, Uzbekistan, but were told they had to leave. The family ended up in Kyrgyzstan, where they worked in the cotton fields near the Uzbeki border.

My father's life began in Dokshitzy, a town 68 miles northeast of Minsk, which at the time was part of the Second Polish Republic. His father died when he was 10 years old, and his mother was left to feed five children on the slim wages of a seamstress. To bring in extra income, my father was sent to work in a relative's bakery in Vilna, where he studied at the Slobodka Yeshiva, until the Rebbe realized he was more interested in Communism than the Talmud. Conscripted into the Polish army, he could not join his family when they emigrated to Palestine in 1935. When the Polish army was defeated at the start of World War II, my father returned to Vilna and then escaped to live with relatives in Illya, Belarus. Until the Germans invaded, life under Russian rule from September 1939 until June 1941 was tranquil. Then, on Purim 1942, the Germans dragged Jews out of their homes to the town square, had them dig a pit, stripped them and shot them so they fell into the mass grave they dug for themselves. By noon the Germans killed 1,500 men, women, and children. Then they poured gasoline over the bodies and set them on fire to get rid of "the evidence."

My father watched the massacre from the attic of the bakery where he worked, and that night escaped into the woods, where he met other Jews who survived because they had special skills needed by the German occupiers. He and a comrade lived like scavengers. Every few nights they knocked on doors of the local farms, hoping to get a bottle of milk and some bread. They foraged for berries and made efforts to join the Belarus partisans, but had little chance to be accepted without guns, especially as Jews.

Preface: Generations of the Holocaust   11

Every night, Ivan Safanov, an acquaintance and righteous gentile, sent his children to bring them food and wash their lice infested clothes. He eventually persuaded the partisans to accept them. My father was valuable to them even without a rifle. During his time in the Polish Army, my father had learned to fix ammunition blindfolded and was an expert saboteur. He received many medals for bombing railroad tracks, and German army stations. Toward the end of the war, he and his fellow partisans joined the Red Army, where he was assigned to the liberating forces as a translator in Berlin.

I can just imagine how heartening it was for my father to be integrated into my mother's family of parents, siblings, and cousins, with celebrations of holidays, marriages and births. My grandfather appreciated how my father prayed and was learned in Jewish texts, and he said to him, "I like how you *daven* (pray), why don't you marry my daughter?"[1]

My mother's family dispersed to Israel and America. My parents opted for Israel because my mother wanted to be with her parents, and my father was eager to reunite with his nuclear family, but tragedy intervened. His brother was killed fighting in Latrun, when they tried to capture Jerusalem during the 1948 War of Independence. Unlike other children of survivors who were named after a relative murdered in the Holocaust, I was named after Aryeh Fagelman. Aryeh is Hebrew for Leibeleh, which means lion, and beloved one, and Haviva, my name, means beloved one.

Leibeleh was looking forward to being reunited with his older brother and wanted to help him acclimate to Israel. The family never got over his death because his body was never found. It is believed his remains were buried in a mass grave on Har Herzl, the military cemetery in Jerusalem.

My Story

With Leibeleh as my namesake and growing up in Israel for the first 10 years of my life, my identity as an Israeli and a Zionist were forged in steel. Being a child of Holocaust survivors was not part of my consciousness. I was very disheartened to learn that we were moving to America. My uncle George, who came to Israel to find a bride, was appalled at how we were living on a dirt road in a one-room house with a kitchen. We had a spacious back yard

---

1 Emanuella Grinberg. "How the Definition of Holocaust Survivor Has Changed Since the End of World War II", *Smithsonian Magazine,* May 1, 2019.

with fruit trees, a chicken coop, some ducks, and an orange grove a few feet away. But all the trappings of our humble home did not impress him.

My father was very disillusioned with God and religion, as was the rest of his family, with the exception of his mother – who was very pious and lived in Mea Shearim with her second husband, a rabbi of a synagogue and Beit Midrash.

My Jewish identity emerged in the United States when I became cognizant of Christians. I recall often asking new acquaintances, "Are you Christian or Jewish?" I was enrolled in public school, in Borough Park, Brooklyn and attended Talmud Torah in the afternoons. On Saturdays, we were required to go to junior congregation. I became congregation president, excelled in the classroom, koshered my house for Passover, instituted the family's Friday night Shabbat ritual and meal. I sat next to my father for Rosh Hashana and Yom Kippur, enveloped in his *tallit* (prayer shawl) as he taught me how pray. As I got older, I had to sit next to my mother and the rest of the women in their section of the Orthodox synagogue.

The shock of learning about the persecution of Jews came when we visited relatives and I was flipping through a coffee table book with pictures of heaps of dead bodies. I don't recall asking any questions. Also, one of my mother's cousins, Herschele, from her hometown, lost his wife and children in "The War," *der milchume*. He never remarried and lived with his brother and his family. Every summer when I visited them for a few days in Brighton Beach, Herschele would always greet me with a smile. I knew of his loss but was given no details.

My awareness intensified, but still felt amorphous until I met Dina Rosenfeld, on the first day of seventh grade. She was born in Rumania to parents who each lost their spouses and children during the Holocaust. Her father was imprisoned after the war for political beliefs and died of a heart attack soon after he was released. Dina's mother had a number on her arm, and visits to their apartment evoked loss and mourning.

Dina and I made an effort to Americanize. We joined the local chapter of B'nai B'rith Youth Organization (BBYO), and I became president. We got involved in volunteer activities such as selling chocolates for a cause, and we were candy stripers at the local Maimonides Hospital. We went to summer camp and became very active in our respective high schools. My father was not pleased with the BBYO because it was not Zionist. I got involved in regional activities as co-chair – with a fellow child of Holocaust survivors – of the Jewish heritage committee. We only discovered the daughters of survivors' part of our identities later in our lives.

My father's family in America was more assimilated than we were. His father had immigrated to the United States around 1907 and brought along a sister and brother. When my grandfather sent a beardless picture of himself back home to Dokshitzy, my great-grandfather warned his daughter not to join her husband in America because "you cannot be Jewish in America." After five years my grandfather went back to Europe and had two more children. In the United States, my father's cousins became lawyers, dentists and two became leading literary critics: Alfred Kazin and Pearl Kazin Bell. At age 11 in 1960, I was not aware of the publication of Elie Wiesel's *Night*, nor of Alfred's Kazin's book review of *Night*, a review that catapulted the book to major heights. The two of them appeared on many panels in academic circles. To me, they were just cousins with book-lined apartments on the Upper West Side of Manhattan. Pearl spoke Yiddish, which enabled her to converse with my parents. Alfred introduced me to lox and bagels from Zabars for Sunday brunch, which was the extent of his *ersatz* Jewish observance.

In a public high school in the 1960s, a world history textbook contained one paragraph mentioning six million Jews were murdered during World War II. My consciousness of the details behind that huge number began to emerge as my sister and I went shopping with my mother on the Lower East Side of Manhattan – where many of the store owners were Holocaust survivors with numbers tattooed on their arms. Conversations between my mother and the shop keepers always led to talking about *der milchume*.

During my college years, the systematic annihilation of European Jewry sunk in when I heard a lecture presented by Rabbi Yitz Greenberg at Yale University. However, my personal identity was still focused on Israel, particularly after the Six-Day War in June 1967, and on solidifying a more spiritual Jewish life for myself. I wanted to volunteer during the Six-Day War, but I needed my parents' permission to be accepted and that was not forthcoming. The following year I returned to Israel for the first time, and it would be the first of countless trips.

The feminist movement was in the air, and we Jewish women who were engaged in Jewish life realized that the consciousness raising that was prevalent at the time did not fully speak to us. I attended Brooklyn College in the late 1960s, a time when the feminist movement on campus and Black consciousness were catalysts for me to think about my Jewish identity. The feminists and radicals on campus were intellectually stimulating, involved as they were in the nationwide anti-Vietnam War campaign, and in anti-establishment political causes. These groups, however, were unintelligently hostile towards their Judaism and the State of Israel.

In 1971, I was one of the 10 women who participated in the first Jewish feminist group, Ezrat Nashim. We shared our personal experiences growing up as Jewish women, we studied Jewish texts and Talmud, to learn what was law and what was social custom regarding certain religious practices – such as saying Kiddush at a Shabbat meal. I was one of the organizers of the First Jewish Feminist Conference in New York in February 1973.[2]

Developing an Identity as a Child of Holocaust Survivors

By then I was living in Boston and was instrumental in establishing a Jewish feminist conscious-raising group there, one that still meets. Now, with Covid-19, we meet monthly on Zoom. I met Bella Savran, a fellow daughter of Holocaust survivors who was a social worker in that group. We got together with some academic psychologists who wanted to explore what Jewish text had to teach us about psychotherapy.

This was also when I was studied family therapy. One assignment was to act out a non-verbal movement representation of our family, called sculpture. When I portrayed my family, my teacher Fred Duhl commented, "Your father is a survivor." I never thought of him that way, I always envisioned my father as a partisan. That remark was etched in my mind and shifted my identity from being a Jewish feminist to include being a daughter of Holocaust survivors. Also, when I had to prepare my family genealogy, I realized, for the first time, how many branches were missing from the family tree.

Then, in the spring of 1975 *Response: A Contemporary Jewish Review*, published a special issue devoted to *The Holocaust: Our Generation Looks Back*. The journal included a discussion between five children of Holocaust survivors (a few whom I knew, among them Dina Rosenfeld). Bella and I commented to each other, "Ha, Ha! This is a beginning of a group."

The idea for an awareness group for children of Holocaust survivors came to us because of our experience with the Jewish feminist group. The opportunity to be with other Jewish feminists reduced our isolation and gave Jewish women a voice in the sea of feminists. The parallel for us was that children of Holocaust survivors who felt different from their American Jewish peers could benefit from meeting each other, share family

---

2   Elizabeth Koltun, ed., *The Jewish Woman: New Perspectives*, New York: Schocken Books, 1976.

Preface: Generations of the Holocaust   15

backgrounds, and explore how one's current life has been influenced by this family background.

As luck would have it, when we approached Rabbi Joseph Polak[3] of Boston University Hillel, he was very receptive to the idea because he was an infant survivor of the Holocaust. Born in Holland, he survived Westerbork and Bergen-Belsen with his mother, who vowed they would become religious if they survived. And so it was.

In the fall of 1975, we posted flyers for awareness groups for children of Holocaust survivors around the university campus and in Jewish stores in Brookline. We interviewed prospective members and ended up with two groups, each to last for eight sessions. These groups were a catalyst that allowed members to feel a camaraderie and normalize life experiences they thought were extreme in their own families; to support each other to communicate with their parents, and to mourn relatives they never knew.[4]

We understood that a historical trauma necessitated a communal mourning experience. Along with Moshe Waldoks,[5] we approached Rabbi Yitz Greenberg to organize a conference for children of Holocaust survivors under the auspices of his organization, Holocaust Resource Center of the National Jewish Center for Learning and Leadership. He was excited about the idea and told us to wait until funds became available.

In the meantime, I learned that a group of psychoanalysts at the American Psychoanalytic Association had finally convinced the leaders in the organization to permit a Group for the Psychoanalytic Study of the Effect of the Holocaust on the Second Generation. I was welcomed with open arms to attend the annual meetings because the members were interested in what I was learning from my participants in the short-term awareness groups. That was when the term Second Generation (2Gs) was coined to describe the sons and daughters of Holocaust survivors, a name that has

---

3 Joseph Polak, *After the Holocaust the Bells Still Ring*, New York: Urim Publications, 2015.
4 Eva Fogelman, "Awareness Groups for Children of Holocaust Survivors", *Jewish Advocate*, Dec. 29, 1977: 3; Eva Fogelman, "Awareness Groups for Children of Holocaust Survivors", *Shoah: A Review of Holocaust Studies and Commemorations*, 4 (1978), 11; Eva Fogelman and Bella Savran, "Therapeutic Groups for Children of Holocaust Survivors", *International Journal of Group Psychotherapy*, 29 (2) (1979), 211–235.
5 Moshe Waldoks and William Novak, eds., *The Big Book on Jewish Humor*, New York: Harper Collins, 1981. Waldoks is also a historian and a Rabbi.

identified them for decades – and their children are known as Third Generation or 3Gs.

On June 19, 1977, Helen Epstein's watershed article, "Heirs of the Holocaust," was published as a cover story in the Sunday Magazine of the *New York Times* and was read by two million people. Children of survivors stopped being an invisible group in the American landscape to become a loud and visible group in American society. The interviewees articulated what many sons and daughters of survivors felt but could not put into words. The article discussed the groups that Savran and I led, which spurred others to start similar groups in other parts of the country.

That summer, I visited my birthplace on my way to Israel to attend an International Psychoanalytic Association meeting, which held the study group on the Second Generation. I was offered an opportunity to work with the President of the Israeli Psychoanalytic Association, Hillel Klein, to conduct research, to lecture and lead a group for Second Generation at Hebrew University. In Israel in 1978, the mental-health profession was still in denial about the Holocaust influencing the emotional lives of the survivors' offspring. I was told time and again that I was bringing an American phenomenon to Israel. The only difference that emerges is that sons and daughters of Holocaust survivors who grew up in Israel did not feel alienated or different from their peers, unlike their cohorts in America.

When Helen Epstein's book, *Children of the Holocaust: Conversations with Sons and Daughters of Survivors*, was published in the spring of 1979, it continued to spark interest in this population, which was eager to explore the effects of growing up with survivor parents. Rabbi Greenberg procured the funds for a conference, and asked Savran and me to organize it in the fall. We invited a few others to work with us, and Greenberg's organization would do all the logistical work.

Organizing the Second Generation Movement

Without much lead time we gathered 600 children of survivors for the First National Conference on Children of Holocaust Survivors, November 4, 1979, in New York City. What we learned is that Second Generation was a group of highly functioning Baby Boomers who resented being scrutinized by so-called experts for signs of psychopathology. The conference took on a different tone when Second Generation members spoke for themselves.

The two-day event ended with a memorial service led by theologian, historian and rabbi, Michael Berenbaum, whose remarks acknowledged the rifts between Second Generation and the psychologists and psychiatrists, religious differences that came up, arguments about the definition of Second Generation and child survivors, and the focus for the future – the question of whether there be social action groups or what was referred to as rap groups. Berenbaum told the audience we were all bound together by horrific, historical events that broke our hearts, and to lay those differences aside. It was time to say Kaddish.

The conference closed with remarks from Rabbi Greenberg, who summed it all up by saying "the secret of our strength is when we come together." Six candles were lit – a liturgical moment symbolizing the memory of the Holocaust. Greenberg explained: "whether it is a symbol of *yorzeit* candle because obviously we mourn and remember, or lighting candle against the darkness…. or it is the flames of Auschwitz which burn us up and burn up our tradition." He concluded with the Kaddish prayer for the millions who have no one to say Kaddish for them. And then the audience burst into song of the last words of the Kaddish, "He will make peace on us and on all of Israel."

The participants, who came from all over the United States, a few from abroad, returned to their hometowns and started organizations and groups. Most notable was work done by Jeanette Friedman, who organized a meeting in Teaneck, NJ to create a social action organization to promote Holocaust education and fight local antisemitism. That group motivated local clerics of all religions, politicians from both parties, and even Governor Tom Kean, who formed a state commission to promote Holocaust Education in New Jersey schools. While it took time, New Jersey was one of the first states to make Holocaust Education mandatory.

The Fall of 1979 changed my professional identity. I enrolled in a doctoral program to study Social and Personality Psychology with Stephen P. Cohen, an expert in group dynamics and the Middle East conflict, and with Stanley Milgram, known for his studies on disobedience to authority. Being a psychoanalytic psychotherapist and learning family systems had provided me with limited tools for understanding human beings' behavior in extreme situations and their aftermaths.

Uncovering conscious and unconscious motivations was not sufficient. I was becoming a social psychologist to study what differentiates myths, anecdotes, and systematic research. What does the larger society have to do with the development of certain myths about a group? Why did Holocaust survivors and their families continue to be "the other" in American and Israeli societies?

I started asking questions most psychoanalysts avoid: How does being a member of a victimized group influence one's identity religiously, ethnically, and culturally? What is the quality of communications between the generations when there is a taboo about talking about a subject that is avoided at all costs? How are relationships established when lack of trust is a major concern? What are the commonalities and differences among Second Generation? What are the group dynamics in a group of Second Generation people? Do they replicate the dynamics found in survivor families?

A core group of survivors and Second Generation in New York was mobilized by the organizers of the World Gathering of Holocaust Survivors. They set up a day-long program for the more than 1,000 young adults who accompanied their parents (or came alone) to Israel in June 1981, exploring everything from how the American Second Generation relates to Israel and how the Israeli Second Generation relates to America. This event was a turning point for the Second Generation. They pledged to continue Holocaust commemoration and education.

The most memorable moment of this huge event for me was when Israeli poet, Rivka Miriam, spoke to our generation and said, "We Israelis are the actors on a stage and you are the audience. We are tired of being the actors." In today's parlance, she saw all Jews in the Diaspora as privileged.

At the Gathering, I embarked on my study of why non-Jews risked their lives to save Jews during the Holocaust, and it became my doctoral dissertation. In 1986, Rabbi Harold Schulweis and I co-founded the Jewish Foundation for Christian Rescuers (The Jewish Foundation for the Righteous). We eventually provided financial and social support to 1,600 rescuers in 26 countries and organized several academic conferences at Princeton University and elsewhere.

After the World Gathering, even without the internet and WhatsApp, we formed an International Network of Children of Jewish Holocaust Survivors. We had our own conferences and educational panels, and we accompanied the survivors to the American Gatherings in Washington, DC and Philadelphia. In 1984 our Second Generation conference in New York attracted 1,600 attendees, and the panelists were all outstanding scholars in their respective fields. A documentary film, *Breaking the Silence: The Generation After the Holocaust*, which I wrote and co-produced, was shown nationally on PBS, and that, too, gave the Second Generation movement gravity as well as "buzz." A core group of the network met a few times a year in different cities. We organized conferences in California and one in Israel.

The active members in local organizations around the United States and abroad got involved to solidify local Holocaust commemorations, to build a few Holocaust museums and monuments, to lobby for mandatory

Holocaust education in local states, to provide social support to aging Holocaust survivors, to take roots trips to Europe, to lecture, and to engage in other creative projects.

Clearly, the Second Generation movement brought like-minded people together because of their shared purpose and their desire to make a difference in their local communities. Those who needed emotional support were able to form self-help groups or groups with a trained leader. To fulfill the latter goal, one had to live in a larger city to find a core group. The groups with leaders continued to be in vogue in the 1980s and early 1990s.

Leaderless groups often fizzled when a conflict erupted in the group and could not be resolved. Sometimes they dissolved when people felt the group served its purpose, and it was time for them to move on.

In New York City, one child of Holocaust survivors who started a group every evening of the week, suddenly decided he had enough and abruptly ended his groups without a termination process. I have continued to lead a weekly psychoanalytic group for more than 30 years with one original member in New York City.

With the evolution of the computer age, many group meeting in people's living rooms or clinicians' offices migrated online, where Second Generation people from all over the world were able to connect – from the US and Israel, to Canada, the UK and even Australia.

The List and Other 2G Groups Connect Online

In the early 1990s it began with mailing lists, Shamash, a Jewish email List that served as a vehicle to enable offspring of survivors to connect with each other. One person would start a discussion on email relevant to being a child of Holocaust survivors, such as, did your parents allow you to go on school trips? A chain dialogue would start and continue until a new topic was raised. All the previous exchanges were visible. The early interaction on the email List focused on comparing psychological effects of growing up in a Holocaust survivor family. The participants tended to be those who felt different from their American Jewish peers, questioned how their parents and other relatives communicated their horrific ordeals to them – if they did, at all – and struggled with their identity as Second Generation from shame to pride; those who overly identified with the victimization, and those searched for support to overcome survivor's guilt.

Conflicts in these internet discussions revolved around certain participants being angry with those who blamed their survivor parents for everything that was wrong in their lives. Those who might have benefitted from more professional help for their psychological challenges were not eager to engage in a therapeutic relationship. Courage is needed to engage in psychotherapeutic relationships and work through emotional problems, instead of complaining to your peers about the same issues over and over again.

These online email conversations had monitors who vetted what was emailed to everyone on The List. At times participants were so vitriolic, their messages were not posted. Monitors burned out when they constantly had to intervene to negotiate conflicts too many times. In retrospect, the anger expressed in these online groups is not a surprising outcome. A tendency exists for people with a common background of victimization to end up expressing anger at each other because the common enemy is absent. Psychologically speaking, this is the metaprocess of these groups in real life and online.

In the mid-1990s, America OnLine, precursor to AOL, had forums online which allowed Second Generation people from across America to message each other. Because airline flights in those days were reasonable, participants often visited each other. When the conflicts in the group became too intense, some people left the discussions and formed new groups. A core group of women who met at the Holocaust Scholar's conference in Oxford, in 2000, formed Cyberfluffies on Yahoo, and continued discussions on women's issues such as weight problems, and a desire to make a difference in the world. "Remember/Zachor" was their watchword. And after that came, "Watch your diet!"

In many of these online Second Generation groups, participants became aware of commonalities as well as differences. But the ugly game, The Suffering Olympics, always came into play. Who suffered more? And the more your parents suffered, the more authentic a 2G you were. In initial group discussions, the hierarchy of suffering was an attempt to determine who belongs and who does not belong in these groups. Second Generation whose parents were in concentration camps did not want to accept those whose parents were flee cases, in hiding or passing as gentiles. It mattered not to the "hard core" that parents who fled lost their homes, country, possessions, family members. The other controversial criteria for membership focused on whether to allow Second Generation offspring of mixed marriages with non-Jewish descendants, or children of non-Jewish parents who suffered Nazi German persecution, to join the dialogue. While an insignificant percentage of Jewish Holocaust survivors married non-Jews (a few converted, others did not), the resentment against children of mixed marriages, especially between Germans and Jews, was not a nice thing to see.

Unlike face-to-face groups, in many online groups there are participants who post their feelings and ideas regularly, while others "lurk," a term from the first days of the internet, where people read and do not respond. These silent members are curious about what it was like growing up with Holocaust survivor parents. They silently identify with some of the more vocal members and find it therapeutic without having to share their own experiences. Hearing others articulate what one is feeling is helpful in the same way readers of Helen Epstein's book found it therapeutic to read about how other members of the Second Generation felt and thought. Verbalization of these aftermaths of the Holocaust in traumatic families provides readers with the vocabulary to articulate their own experiences, which might not have been possible for them before.

With the proliferation of Holocaust-related programs world-wide, several list serves began to disseminate information. The most well-known among them is Generations of the Shoah International/GSI. In recent years the group added a book review section. Another site, AllGenerations, announces upcoming Holocaust-related events, and asks new members to introduce themselves by sharing their family history. Through this process, some people have found missing relatives, affinity groups like *landmanshaften*, and shared displaced persons camp experiences. They also have found family members who survived the Holocaust in similar locales.

Facebook has facilitated dozens of Second and Third Generation groups and some mixed groups, which are local, national or international. There are groups for Holocaust Education and Holocaust Programs for teachers and others. Some groups are open to whoever wants to post and join. Other groups are closed and have criteria that are vetted by their Facebook administrators. Like in the old days of Shamash, it is not uncommon for people who are disgruntled by comments or the control of the administrator to start their own groups.

With the proliferation of these Facebook groups, the panorama of the diversity among the children of Holocaust survivors can be observed. Most blatant, of course, are the political differences. As in American society in general, the divide between right and left political views is so potent that discourse is almost non-existent – but there is burning rage, one side against the other. The American Jewish community is also divided by political ideologies regarding Israel. To the chagrin of established Jewish leadership and "legacy" organizations, most young Jews do not even have Israel on their radar. Whether it is American politics, Middle East politics, antisemitism, or important human rights issues, descendants of Holocaust survivors each feel their political views have been influenced by their parents' persecution as Jews.

To avoid the political divide, one Facebook group, Descendants of Holocaust Survivors (2G Greater NY),[6] a closed group, asks potential participants to agree not to post political comments. It is not always possible to stay away from politics since confrontation with the Holocaust evokes emotions and thoughts that are inevitably political. A recent example is the Polish government's restriction on academic freedom historians who write about Poland and the Holocaust. Another is that American Jews passionate about Israel are moved to speak up for what they believe in, often with painful, insulting results.

The endless game of the Suffering Olympics was solved by people who decided only concentration camp or death camp survivors count, so they created a separate Facebook group for Second Generation who parents survived the camps. No others need apply.

For children of survivors who live in isolated areas, where there are no opportunities to meet others from a similar background, Facebook has been a blessing. It has enabled these individuals to break out of isolation and gain validation for their thoughts and feelings, while learning their upbringing was not so strange.

Realizing that a Holocaust family background is an important part of one's being happens at different times in one's development. Some only discover and acknowledge this aspect of their identity in their older years, in their 60s and 70s. Others were on the young side of the spectrum and were not alive or very young in the mid- to late 1970s when Epstein's book and the First Conference on Children of Holocaust Survivors took place in New York City.

Until recently, I was not involved in any Facebook groups. In 2018, when a Second Generation group started meeting in a 2G's living room in Manhattan, they realized the space was becoming too small for the number of participants who wanted to meet each other. I was asked to help launch the group into a public arena and led a few programs. We used Facebook to promote events and participants started posting comments of mutual interest. With the increase of Facebook followers, Ellen Bachner Greenberg and Jerome Kowalski organized a day conference at the Museum of Jewish Heritage. As with many of these groups, a rift occurred, and an off-shoot group was formed. I was asked to co-found the Facebook group,

---

6   I founded the group together with Ellen Bachner Greenberg.

Descendants of Holocaust Survivors (2G Greater New York). To differentiate ourselves from other groups, we opted for a closed group devoid of politics. We wanted to be inclusive and bring together concerns that unite us, not what separates us.

When I started perusing the world of descendants of Holocaust survivors on Facebook, I was overwhelmed by the dozen or so groups that exist. Many serve the purpose of memorializing our beloved parents and grandparents who died, sharing historical information that is new or is significant for a specific date. Of course, events of interest are highlighted and links to participate are posted.

During the pandemic that brought normal life to a halt in the United States in March 2020, people's lives became more isolated. Facebook for descendants of Holocaust survivors became more significant. I led a special session for members of 2G Greater NY about the effects of Facebook on the psychological impact of Covid-19 specific to Second Generation. Participants asked questions and shared their thoughts. Those who needed to continue the discussion found supportive contacts. I participated in a similar event with Gaby Glassman, a 2G leader with a group in England on Zoom.

With Zoom, descendants of Holocaust survivors on Facebook groups availed themselves of the new technology and began to broadcast commemorations, scholarly panels and discussion groups on. Facebook was used to advertise and promote these events which were intellectually stimulating, emotionally gratifying, and most importantly, reduced the sense of isolation that is so prevalent during the pandemic – particularly for people who live alone or away from family and friends. Some of the 2G groups, in Hartford Connecticut (Voices of Hope), Washington DC (The Generation After), among others, continue to present programs on Zoom.

One group that stands out for reaching out internationally and for innovative programming is 3GNY. Their Facebook page has attracted more than 8,000 participants worldwide. They have co-sponsored programs with Israel, England, Canada, and that are recorded and archived online. 3GNY has a training program to teach grandchildren of Holocaust survivors to tell their grandparents' stories in classrooms (WEDU). Facebook enables them to reach out to perspective members to sign up to take the class. I also led an 8-week group on Zoom through 3GNY called Love & Sex Across Holocaust Generations. The 3GNY Facebook link brought participants together from the United States and Israel.

My personal preference has always been to meet with people directly or speak on the phone. What initially turned me off to Facebook was a patient who found out that her boyfriend jilted her on Facebook. She would look at his page daily to learn about his new girlfriend from pictures he was posting. After a few months of therapy, she finally weaned herself off his Facebook and blocked him. She was not the only one who suffered from what she saw on Facebook or was blocked from someone's Facebook. The silly items people posted, such as what they ate for breakfast was another turn off.

I was not a joiner of any of the early email groups, nor of Facebook. I did join AllGenerations because I knew the moderator, I appreciated learning what programs were available so I could share with others and was happy to read family histories from different countries by people who wanted to connect with others from a Holocaust background. AllGenerations was not a vehicle for cross communication.

The 2G Facebook group discussions that I heard about were a mixed bag. On the one hand, it was a medium for 2Gs to disclose the details of growing up with Holocaust survivors and its impact on them. On the other hand, some participants became belligerent to members who expressed blame towards their survivor parents. But then I would hear about people being thrown off Facebook groups because other participants did not like what they had to say, or because they were cruel in their remarks to others.

When I read about Judy Baumel-Schwartz because her father's Shofar was on display at the Auschwitz Exhibit at the Museum of Jewish Heritage, I stumbled across "The List" that was rooted in the far past and asked if I might join. It seemed that people were supportive of each other. I soon realized many of these people had known each other for almost 30 plus years. Whether they met each other in person or not, the interactions among the members felt like a family. They had been together through losses, births, illnesses, and celebrations. When a member of The List posts a tragedy, they feel less alone. Knowing that others care, even though, they are not physically there to help, is emotionally supportive.

These days descendants of Holocaust survivors who want to connect with others have an array of choices. One can follow postings on Facebook groups for survivors, Second Generation, all generational groups of descendants or Holocaust Education and social action groups. For those of us in cities with many others with the same kind of background, companionship through Facebook is a way to avoid more intimate social interaction. Descendants who live in rural or more isolated areas, find it worthwhile to connect with others who understand them in ways that do not have to be explained.

Yes, there are many differences between us, but a certain familiarity can override the differences. Unfortunately, in recent years, the political divide among descendants of Holocaust survivors in the United States and differences in attitudes towards the Israeli government, has severed interaction between various factions. The comments posted on Facebook have been vicious. Some participants have removed themselves from these groups and few others formed groups that allow them to express and act on their political ideologies.

Facebook as a medium for social interaction is being extensively studied. Overall findings suggest a "Facebook paradox,"[7] meaning it can be helpful or harmful to well-being, and it is, unfortunately, mostly negative. Social connection through Facebook or other internet connections cause stress, anxiety, and depression, boost or destroy self-worth, provide comfort and joy, or cause rage. The posts can prevent loneliness, especially in old age.

On the other hand, Facebooking is "negatively linked to users' psychological well-being through online social relationship satisfaction, perceived social support, and social interaction anxiety."[8]

"The psychological well-being of introverted users depends more heavily upon perceived social support which appears stronger for introverts than for extraverts. Online and online social contexts can complement and reinforce each other. On the one hand, fostering online social relationships on Facebook can expand users' social network, accumulate social capital, prompt users to engage actively in social groups, and promote self-presentation. All of these outcomes may benefit online social relationships via obtaining richer information, facilitating deeper social interactions, and boosting self-efficacy. On the other hand, reinforcing online social relationships enables individuals to obtain intimacy, interpersonal trust, and strong social ties. This, in turn, may help Facebook users maintain more meaningful and closer social relationships in online social contexts."[9]

With the proliferation of Facebook groups initiated by descendants of Holocaust survivors, research on participants and non-participants in these groups can enhance our understanding of its usefulness as a medium for this population and other historically traumatized groups.

The List and its longevity and evolution is a unique presence in the age of the internet. One might think of it today as having long distance phone calls

---

7   Xiaomeng Hu, Andrew Kim, Nicholas Siwek and David Wilder, "The Facebook Paradox: Effects of Facebooking on Individuals' Social Relationships and Psychological Well-Being", *Front. Psychol.*, January 31, 2017 | https://doi.org/10.3389/fpsyg.2017.00087
8   "The Facebook Paradox", ibid.
9   "The Facebook Paradox", ibid.

replaced by WhatsApp. The personal relationships formed over the years contributes to the emotional connections that are missing in the current Facebook groups that many descendants of Holocaust survivors are now joining. Looking forward to the future, there needs to be a link between online and offline interactions among descendants of Holocaust survivors. There is nothing like getting together for a cup of coffee.

Prof. Judith Tydor Baumel-Schwartz
Introduction

It is 7:00 am in Israel on a chilly winter morning. Shivering as I get out of bed, I zip up my floor length velour robe and turn on my computer, waiting for it (and me) to warm up. When it finally does, I pry my eyes open to scan my email, checking what has gone on in the world while I slept. Running my eyes down the length of my inbox, I delete message after message until I reach one of three kinds: work-related, family news, or those from "The List".

Located all over the globe, members of "The List" are often quite active during the hours I am in bed. On most days, The List spans "only" 10 time zones, but it can sometimes reach 17. When it is 7:00 am where I live, our effervescent Australians have already been up and active for 7 hours, while our lively West Coasters, 10 hours behind me, are winding down, having finished a full day of adventure that I already left behind. By the time I lift my eyes from the screen after responding to List discussions that began, or continued, while I slept, an hour has often passed. To remain an active family member often takes time and patience; the same holds true when trying to remain an active member of our online Second Generation "family".

This is a book about an online community of the Second Generation (2g), children of Holocaust survivors. But it is also about the First Generation, our parents, their experiences, and how those experiences affected us. "In the beginning there was Auschwitz", writes Second Generation author and literary critic Melvin J. Bukiet, reminding us how much of the where, when, and to whom we were born, had been determined by the Holocaust. "On the most literal level, their fathers would not have met their mothers if not for the huge dislocations that thrust the few remnants of European Jewry into contact with spouses they would never have otherwise encountered except for DP camps or in the twentieth-century Diaspora. The Second Generation's very existence is dependent on the whirlwind their parents barely escaped".[1] The locus of this book is therefore the area of an equilateral

---

1 Melvin J. Bukiet, *Nothing Makes You Free: Writings By Descendants of Jewish Holocaust Survivors*, New York and London: W. W. Norton and Company, 2002: 13.

triangle, created by the interaction of its three sides: The First Generation, the Second Generation, and the Holocaust.

There is little doubt that the Holocaust was a watershed event of the 20th century. Even as it occurred, scholars were already studying its causes and various aspects of its development. During the first decades after the war's end, they focused upon what they felt were its various major facets: Nazi policy towards the Jews, Jewish leadership, resistance, rescue attempts, and the Nazi camp universe. By the 1970s, academic scholarship about the Holocaust had expanded to include social and cultural topics, such as daily life under Nazi rule, the plight of refugees, and the fate of children under the Nazis. All were treated as worthy research topics that helped us better understand the dynamics of this catastrophic period.

As time passed, new fields of research developed, including those pertaining to descendants of Holocaust survivors – the "Second Generation" ("2g"), and later the "Third Generation" ("3g"). Initial studies of these groups were primarily sociological and psychological.[2] Eventually, studies of the 2gs and 3gs began to emerge in other disciplines – sociology, communications, law, literature, film – and more recently in biological and medical fields including the epigenetics of inherited trauma, or 2g and 3g health issues.[3]

Today, new books about the descendants of Holocaust survivors are often multi-disciplinary[4] or focus on specific topics such as those who choose particular professions.[5] Others, such as this volume, target specific 2g and 3g

---

2 See, for example: Arie Nadler, Sophie Kav-Venaki and Beny Gleitman, "Transgenerational Effects of the Holocaust: Externalization of Aggression in Second Generation of Holocaust Survivors", *Journal of Consulting and Clinical Psychology*, 53(3) (1985), 365–369.

3 For example: Victoria Aarons and Alan L. Berger, *Third Generation Holocaust Representation: Trauma, History, and Memory*, Evanston, IL: Northwestern University Press, 2017; Liat Steir-Livny, "Growing Up in the Shadow of the Past: Second Generation Holocaust Survivors' Childhoods as Depicted in Israeli Documentary Films", in: Anat Helman (ed.), *No Small Matter: Features of Jewish Childhood, Studies in Contemporary Jewry* 32 (2021): 157–168; Natan P. F. Kellerman, "Epigenetic Transmission of Holocaust Trauma: Can Nightmares Be Inherited?", *Israeli Journal of Psychiatry Related Science* 50(1) (2013): 9–33.

4 Judith Tydor Baumel-Schwartz and Amit Shrira, *Routledge International Handbook of Multidisciplinary Perspective on Descendants of Holocaust Survivors*, (Routledge, forthcoming 2023).

5 Judith Tydor Baumel-Schwartz and Shmuel Refael, *Researchers Remember: Research as an Arena of Memory for Descendants of Holocaust Survivors*,

groups, in this case, those who formed a transnational, English-speaking, online Second Generation Community that has continued to exist for over a quarter of a century.

How It All Began

The List was not the first 2g organization to be founded, although it was possibly the first 2g online group of its kind. The first documented 2g groups were actually short-term awareness groups, run by psychologists Bella Savran and Dr. Eva Fogelman at Boston University (1976), and then by Fogelman at the Hebrew University of Jerusalem (1978).[6] Their inspiration came from reading what they felt was an eye opening dialogue between children of survivors that had been published in *Response: A Contemporary Jewish Review*, in 1975. Meeting for 8 to 12 sessions, these were the first 2g groups that were formed to discuss issues pertaining to the lives of children of survivors.

Interest in the Holocaust reached unparalleled heights following the broadcast of NBC's 1978 docudrama of that name,[7] and the publication of Helen Epstein's path-breaking 2g introspection, *Children of the Holocaust*. Bringing the topic of Holocaust survivors' offspring to the forefront,[8] the first 2g gatherings soon began to crystallize, one in the United States and the other Israel. In November 1979 the First Conference of the Second Generation, held at Hebrew Union College, laid the groundwork for a 2g organization that would be established a year and a half later, following the World Gathering of Jewish Holocaust Survivors held in Jerusalem in June 1981.[9] Although it was called "The International Network of Children of Jewish Holocaust Survivors" (INCJHS), it soon became a primarily American organization, headed by 2g activist and lawyer, Menachem Rosensaft, son

---

A Collected Volume of Academic Autobiographies, Bern: Peter Lang Publishers, 2021.
6 Author's correspondence with Dr. Eva Fogelman, July 18, 2021; Author's correspondence with Helen Epstein, July 16, 2021.
7 *Holocaust*, written by Gerald Green, directed by Marvin J. Chomsky, April 16–19, 1978, https://www.imdb.com/title/tt0077025/, retrieved on August 11, 2021.
8 Helen Epstein, *Children of the Holocaust*, New York: Putnam, 1979.
9 Jeanette Friedman, "Rabbi 'Yitz' Greenberg at 80: A Paradigm Changer", *Jewishlink*, June 27, 2013. https://jewishlink.news/features/1000-rabbi-yitz-greenberg-at-80-a-paradigm-changer, retrieved on August 11, 2021.

of post-war activists Josef and Dr. Hadassah Bimko-Rosensaft, a founding member of the United States Holocaust Memorial Council.

The first Israeli initiative to establish a 2g organization actually predated the American one. In March 1980, having heard about the American 2g conference, historian Judy Tydor Baumel (later Schwartz), and psychodrama specialist Ya'akov Naor, founded the *Irgun Yaldei Nitzolei Shoah Beyisrael* – The Israeli Organization for Children of Holocaust Survivors, a long-named, short-lived body which lasted for less than six months because of discord over its organizational focus. Should its forty or so members devote their energies to hashing out personal fallout from their 2g background, or should they use that time to volunteer among elderly or indigent survivors? Could they do both? Unable to reach a consensus, even between the organizers, the group disbanded a year before the establishment of its American counterpart. Nevertheless, it heralded the creation of a larger Israeli 2g organization, *Irgun Dor Hemshech Limoreshet Hashoah VeHagevurah* (Second Generation Organization for the Legacy of Holocaust and Heroism) which, like the INCJHS, was also – unsurprisingly – formed in the wake of the 1981 World Gathering in Jerusalem. "The Second Generation will never know what the First Generation does in its bones, but what the Second Generation knows better than anyone else is the First Generation", writes Bukiet.[10] When survivors gather, their children are rarely far behind.

It was not by chance that both the American and the Israeli 2g national organizations were catalyzed by a Holocaust survivor conference and supported or partially initiated by survivor organizations with organizational clout and financial resources. In Israel, leaders of the "Partisans, Underground, and Ghetto Resistance Fighters Organizations" such as Bela-Elster-Rotenberg ("Wanda"), Ya'akov Greenstein, Stefan Grayek, and Moshe Kalchheim, initiated the creation of *Irgun Dor Hemshech,* while Ya'akov Zilberstein, head of the Organization of Former Nazi Prisoners, financially assisted the organization at various early junctures. In the United States, Benjamin Meed, president of the "American Gathering of Jewish Holocaust Survivors" and one of the founders of WAGRO, the Warsaw Ghetto Resistance Organization (1963),[11] was very active in spearheading the American initiative.

---

10 Bukiet, *Nothing Makes You Free,* p. 14.
11 https://www.jta.org/1963/02/19/archive/warsaw-ghetto-resistance-organization-formed-in-u-s-by-ex-members, retrieved on August 16, 2021.

Are "initiated" and "active", synonyms for "controlling"? It all depends on who one asks. Finances are the "make or break" of many active organizations and, 2g bodies often suffered from chronic deficits. Thus, the backing of survivor organizations was at times critical to their continued existence. Inevitably, the interconnection between survivors and 2g groups led to tacit power struggles between survivors wishing to see their legacy continue, and newly formed 2g organizations determined to set their own path. Debates over questions of policy and practice did not always end with hugs and smiles. Similar to those families where children are only considered adults when they reach late middle age, in some places, it took a generational transition for 2gs to finally come into their own.

Members of the "Second Generation" throughout the world may embody similar characteristics, but the same is not true of 2g organizations. At an early stage the American and Israeli 2g endeavors took on different trajectories, influenced by geography and organizational culture. The sheer geographical vastness of the United States and a tradition of decentralization encouraged the development of local 2g groups throughout the country. These included groups organized by activists including Jeanette Friedman (New Jersey), Charlie Silow (Michigan), and others, that flourished in cities such as Atlanta, Cleveland, Detroit, Los Angeles, Miami, New York, Philadelphia, San Francisco, St. Louis, Teaneck, and Washington DC from the mid-1980s onward. Some groups were connected to the INCJHS, while others began as independent discussion groups. There were also 2g groups that began as a section within an existing Holocaust-related organization such as WAGRO, whose members were acutely aware of the aging process, and wished to create reserves for the future.[12]

Second Generation organizations in Israel developed somewhat differently. Being a relatively small country, geographical parameters precluded the need to develop local 2g groups. During the early 1980s the national *Dor Hemshech* organization, whose members met in the greater Tel-Aviv area, included several dozen 2g activists from all over the country such as Gideon Greif, Rafi Cohen-Almagor, Shmuel Refael, Tzippi Kichler, Gadi Barzilai, and Billie Laniado. Some had been approached by Israeli Knesset Ministry and Holocaust survivor Dov Shilansky, others by Moshe Kalcheim and Yaakov Greenstein of the Partisan Organization. As survivors everywhere recognized that their biological clock was ticking, 2g sections were

---

12 Author's correspondence with Dr. Eva Fogelman, July 18, 2021; Author's correspondence with Jeanette Friedman Sieradski, Aug. 17, 2021.

also being formed in Israeli-based survivor organizations and *Landsmanschaften* such as the Organization of Jews from Salonika, The Association of Jews from Bochnia, and the *She'erit Hapletah* – Bergen Belsen Organization in Israel. And just like in America, the relationship between the survivors and 2gs in these frameworks was often fraught with undercurrents, similar to those between survivors and their children everywhere.[13]

The Making of "The List"

So where does The List enter into all of this? As a technologically based undertaking, it was actually a latecomer among the first wave of 2g organizations. Begun in 1995, The List was the brainchild of Paul Foldes, a 2g electrical engineer and consumer attorney turned businessman, who hadn't been able to find a face-to-face 2g group in the Washington DC area where he lived. Knowing that online communities were an opportunity to reach beyond local meetings, he founded The List even before the web existed.[14]

As an internet-based group, The List bypassed a lot of the problems that some of the face-to-face 2g groups had grappled with. Created when internet communication was just beginning for most people outside of the military and the academic world, it was the first to break local and national barriers to become a truly international, English speaking, 2g framework. Unlike any of the existing 2g face-to-face organizations, it also required no funding. Based on a free internet platform, with moderators working on a volunteer basis, its "meetings" mandated no auditoriums or refreshments, while "mailings" were just additional internet messages requiring no postage. For an online 2g community, the medium was not only the message, but the crucial factor ensuring the group's independence. While the "First Generation" was always present as a topic of discussion, its members no longer had to act as sponsors, either administratively or financially. The "Second Generation" had finally come into its own.

There is, however, a trade-off to independence, and The List was no exception. The first issue it faced was the need to find a permanent cyber-home.

---

13 Author's correspondence with Billie Laniado, July 13, 2021; Author's telephone interview with Prof. Shmuel Refael, July 13, 2021; Author's zoom interview with Prof. Rafi Cohen-Almagor, July 19, 2021; Author's correspondence with Dr. Rachel Kolender, July 25, 2021; Author's correspondence with Prof. Gideon Greif, July 29, 2021; Author's telephone interview with Prof. Gadi Barzilai, August 9, 2021.
14 Author's correspondence with Paul Foldes, July 1, 2021.

Requiring a free location to function, The List suffered from platform instability, spending much of its existence migrating from one free platform to another. The original List began on Shamash, the Jewish network that was a service of Hebrew College in Boston. From there it migrated to Smartgroups where it remained for several years. In 2006 it transitioned to Yahoo groups where it functioned for over a decade. When rumors of Yahoo Groups closing down were first heard in 2018, there was a short-lived, unsuccessful attempt to rework The List as a Gmail Group. Returning to Yahoo for another year and a half, The List ultimately migrated to Google Groups during the summer of 2020, four months before Yahoo closed its groups permanently. "We always seem to be refugees whether or not we admit it", wrote a List member during the last move, echoing the feelings of more than one poster.

Another List dilemma stemmed from its composition and active membership. Within two years of its creation, The List included some 150 participants from 4 continents, more than half of whom were active posters. But List growth had a darker side, as it was often accompanied by the ills of internet forums everywhere, such as flame wars, trolling and cyber-bullying. Add some 2g emotional baggage, shake and serve, and you have a recipe for disaster. Unhappy with the group's dynamics, some members decided to leave while others began a back and forth dynamic of leaving and rejoining more than once. Discussions only calmed down after some of the more volatile posters left The List, while those who remained adapted to List culture.

A third complication had to do with List moderation. As both List creator and its first moderator, Paul Foldes spent enormous amounts of time going through messages before allowing them to be posted. Suffering from burnout, in 1999 he left the active management of The List to others, stepping back, then out, and only returning to The List more than two decades later, in 2021. After Foldes left, List moderators changed every few years, until The List transitioned to google groups in 2020 where it became an unmoderated List. This was only possible because over the years, The List had gone through a form of "natural selection" in terms of membership, topics being discussed, and the nature of those discussions. By 2021 fewer than 50 members remained on The List, only half of whom were active posters. Topics were often mundane, and those who posted adhered to an unwritten rule of conduct: try not to disturb the peace, and word your posts so as not to offend other List members. On the most part, it worked.

The final problem had to do with membership. Why did such an active group eventually lose two thirds of its members? "I guess we became boring", wrote one poster in answer to that question. "It's all because of

Facebook", answered another. "We've reached a different point in our lives, particularly as many of our parents are gone, and we don't need to rehash 2g issues anymore", responded a third. As the heated 2g discussions of the group's first decades died down and were replaced by post about the members' everyday lives, and then by long periods of time without posts at all, there were those who asked if The List was still alive. "It certainly is!" was one poster's definitive answer. "Even our discussions about everyday life are heavily affected by our 2g background", stated another. "We may not mention it anymore, but it's always there, lurking in the background."

So Why a Book?

Soon after the last migration to Google Groups, the idea came up to put together a joint List venture. Hearing about a book I was editing about 2g researchers in which another List member was participating, one of the posters wrote in jest: "You are always writing books, so why not write one about us?". "Actually, why not?!" I thought. And so, we were off.

My first thought about the book revolved around its framework – what would be the best way to show how The List acted as a vehicle to help its members cope with the intergenerational transmission of Holocaust trauma? The next was of scope – what topics should be covered to answer this question? The third pertained to form – would it be better for me to write the history of The List, or to have List members write about their experiences in their own words? Having recently edited several volumes of "ego-documents" – the professional term used for focused memoirs – I decided that a book about The List would best be composed of personal accounts written by List members, detailing their family history, personal background, reasons that propelled them to join The List, and what The List adds to their lives.

Why memoirs? As Marion Kaplan reminds us in her introduction *Her Story, My Story?* a volume of memoirs of women who have written about women during the Holocaust:

> "Memoirs have helped scholars to investigate the lives of non-elites since at least the 1970s. Memoirs have revealed individual's self-understandings, fears, and values, and have provided an entrée into unexplored stories. Yet memoirs offer more than individual lives. The essays in this book are personal, they [...] situate the authors within their [...] very private journeys, [giving us]...a sense of the cultural context and the historical moment. These memoirs may surprise us -- contradicting, illuminating, and deepening the accepted stories."

Eventually we decided on 13 chapters, each written by a veteran List member, with a preface by Dr. Eva Fogelman, a List member who is also a writer, filmmaker, world-renown psychological professional, and a pioneer in the treatment of the psychological effects of the Holocaust on survivors and their descendants. Chapter authors include poets, engineers, geriatric specialists, academic lecturers, and professionals in the humanities, social sciences, medical and natural sciences.

And Now, Thanks

Books do not get published on their own. There are, of course, the author, editor, and publisher, but in addition, there are usually various organizations and individuals without whom the book would not have been published. My thanks to the Finkler Institute of Holocaust Research at Bar-Ilan University that incorporated our "List" book in its "Second" and "Third" Generation project, and helped sponsor this book. Thanks also to the Israel and Golda Koshitzky Department of Jewish History and Contemporary Jewry at Bar-Ilan University which also contributed to the book's publication. Special thanks to my dear friend and colleague, Prof. Shmuel Refael Vivante, Dean of the Faculty of Jewish Studies at Bar-Ilan University, who is a never-ending source of encouragement for all of our Holocaust-related endeavors.

Special thanks go to the Production team at Peter Lang Publishers, Bern, Switzerland, and particularly to Dr. Bianca Matzek and Ulrike Döring, for their marvelous professionalism in publishing this book. It is a pleasure to work with them and produce books together!

One more group of people deserves special thanks – our families. Those with whom we live today, or with whom we have lived in a more recent past, may or may not truly understand what it means to be a 2g, but by now, they certainly realize what it means to live with one. Our very unique thanks – if that is even the correct word – goes to our parents, without whom we would not be members of the "Second" Generation. It is a legacy that none of us would have chosen, but we had no choice. It is a legacy that we might have wanted to forget, but were obviously unable to. And it is a legacy that has seeped into our DNA in a way that permeates everything we do, whether we are aware of it or not.

Our final thanks is to The List, or rather to its members in the past and present, all of whom who contributed to The List throughout the years, without whom it would not have continued to exist, and we would not have been able to write this book.

All in all, we are a mixed bag of 2gs, sometimes so different from each other, and yet, so alike. Each of us has our own story, and together we all have the same story. Our parents are Survivors, with a capital "S". We are all children of Survivors, and that is our legacy, along with all other legacies that our parents consciously or unconsciously bequeathed us. That alone gives us an almost imperceptible common denominator which we may or may not express in daily life, but we can also never erase. It is who they are or were, and it is who we are, and will always be. We may talk about it, we may agonize over it, and we may try to ignore it. But at the end it always there, hovering in the background of every List discussion we have, even on the most banal subjects. And that is what this book is all about.

Marilyn Boehm
From the Ashes to a Flame

Introduction

In Los Angeles, where I grew up, ours was the only family that didn't celebrate Christmas. No trees, no decorations, no presents. When I went back to school after Christmas vacation, the other kids showed off their new sweaters and shoes. I lied and told them that I kept my gifts at home.

Something was different about my family. We were Jews in a Christian world. My parents had strong Hungarian accents. Frequently, there were loud, angry arguments between them, rattling the walls, followed by tension and silence. Dad, who worked as a gardener at Park LaBrea Towers, was typically isolated in his bedroom, listening to classical music. Mom took a bus to work the midnight shift at the Revell plant so she could be home during the day with me and my sister, who was three years older than I.

Because of language difficulties, I had to translate for Mom at Back-to-School nights. I was embarrassed by our differences from the other white-bread kids. When Mom kept us out of school for the Jewish holidays, the kids asked me why. I simply changed the subject, or pretended I'd been sick.

Every year, after Christmas, my sister and I snuck out at night and picked branches from the discarded trees in the alleyways. We brought them home, decorating them with cast off bulbs and silver tinsel. I set my dolls around the tree to pretend they could enjoy the holiday. We knew better than to let Mom know about this, sensing that it would upset her.

One year, in our hunt for abandoned trees, I found some sparkly white "snow" strung across a tree. I eagerly gathered it, dreaming of how stunning it would look on our pretend tree. As I walked home, pleased with my find, I felt my fingertips stinging as if I'd been bitten by a bee. I realized that the pain came from the white angel hair, flecked with tiny glass particles, which I threw to the ground. Was I being punished for savoring a Christian holiday, turning my back on our traditions?

That was to be the last secretive Christmas my sister and I celebrated. I finally got up the nerve to question Mom about why we couldn't observe that holiday like everyone else. Her eyes dropped, reflecting anguish, as she quietly said her family had been killed in the Holocaust because they were

Jews. Reveling in a gentile holiday would have been like spitting on their graves.

When much later I asked my parents to tell me about the Holocaust, I was told simply, "It's too horrible to talk about." I spent years wondering what had happened to them and their families in Europe. It became my personal obsession and puzzle to solve.

What and Who I'm Made of

I never met my mother's parents, Julia and Herman Klein. My grandparents. It still hurts to say it. There was one black and white picture of my mother's family that was taken before the war. It had survived, amazingly, because it had been mailed to American relatives. I took the picture, which was torn, faded, and stained, to a photo shop to have it refurbished. Then I framed it, put it up on my wall, and gave Mom a copy.

Looking at the photo, it was clear that Mom's parents were Orthodox Jews. My grandmother wore a *sheitel* (wig) on her head, while my bearded grandfather was dressed in a conservative suit and wore a large hat. They sat somberly, hands crossed over their laps, surrounded by five of their seven children. Two other female children were born after the photo was taken. Mom, then four or five years old, was the only one smiling in the photo.

Mom told me few details about their lives before the war. It was almost as if their lives had no meaning until the Holocaust, the event that shaped the narrative. From what I could gather, my grandparents met and married in a small village in Hungary called Olaszliszka, two hours away from Budapest. My grandparents lived a very humble existence, renting and working in a bread bakery.

As a young girl, my grandmother was adopted and raised by Rabbi Yeshaya Steiner who lived in the town of Bodrogkeresztúr. I don't know why she was sent to live with this rabbi and his family. It's stunning enough to think that an Orthodox little girl would be given a religious education. She later taught Torah studies to Jewish children in Olaszliszka. Although she had no formal education, she counseled the town's inhabitants, both Jew and gentile, on all sorts of legal and medical matters.

My grandfather was apparently the soft touch, a gentle and kind man. He was Mom's favorite parent, and she believes she was his favorite child. Mom explained that he had been sent away to fight in the Austro-Hungarian Army during World War I. When he came home for a short visit, she was conceived. Mom relished telling the story that, while her dad was gone, she was born on top of the bakery's oven.

Mom had little to say about her teen years, other than that on weekends, she and her friends went hiking in the nearby hills. She lit up when mentioning a very rich young man, a "Count" who fell head over heels in love with her and wanted to marry her. I don't think he was a Jew, so the romance could go no further. How times have changed!

I know only the basics about my mother's other siblings. Her oldest sister, Esther, married a man named Resu with whom she had two small sons, Zoltan and Robbie. The next oldest was Fritzi (Frieda), then Manci (Margaret), then Mom, then the only brother, Sandor (Alex), then Itsa (Ilona), then Ada. Apparently, my grandmother was pregnant with an eighth child, which she miscarried upon learning that my grandfather had been taken prisoner by the Russians. My mother sadly reported that the baby was a boy.

As anti-Jewish measures were implemented during the war, my grandparents were no longer able to rent the bakery. To generate income, Fritzi, Manci, Ada, and Mom moved to Budapest to find work. When, Budapest's Jews were ordered to live in ghettoized yellow Star Houses in 1944, Manci, who had worked for the underground, managed to arrange for the sisters to receive Christian identity papers. At the same time, Mom's sister Ilona made contact with an armed resistance group in Yugoslavia, fought the Nazis, and was shot and killed during a heroic battle. I am proud to say that a member of my family died while bravely fighting Nazism during WWII.

On Shavuot, May 28, 1944, the Jews of Olaszliszka, along with 7,000 other Jews from neighboring villages, were rounded up and deported to Auschwitz. All my relatives who had remained in the village, including my grandparents, uncle, aunt, her husband and two children, were gassed. The Nazis were particularly cruel in selecting religious Jewish holidays for deportations and death.

My father's earlier life was even less certain since it was my mother who always did the talking. Apparently, Dad grew up with five siblings in Budapest. When his father, an alcoholic, "died drunk in a gutter" in his early forties, Dad was taken out of school in the third grade and forced to work to help feed the family. While riding a bicycle, he transported movies in canned receptacles to and from local movie theaters.

It has always saddened me to know that he never had a childhood or friends, while assuming adult responsibilities so young. I never heard him utter one bad word about his mother or her choices. To his dying day, he revered his mother almost as much as, or even more than, he loved Mom.

Before he met Mom, he was married to another Jewish woman. In an "action" by the fascist Arrow Cross in Budapest, Dad's first wife was rounded up on a street corner along with other Jews and was shot and killed. Because Mom told the story, I never heard from Dad about how he learned of her death and how it affected him. Also, one of his brothers apparently died in Auschwitz.

My mother survived the war by posing as a gentile, using false Christian papers. Mom hid, first in Budapest as a nanny, and then as a caretaker in a summer home in the Lake Balaton region, a tourist area outside of Budapest. When the Russians overtook Hungary, Mom was captured by Russian soldiers and gang raped. She didn't go into much detail about the experience, and I didn't pursue it. Her body language told me this topic was one that caused her too much pain.

When I asked about my Dad's experiences during the war, as usual, Mom did all the talking. There were times when Dad corrected her, and she argued with him. "Irene," he'd say, "I was there." Still she argued! That was so typical of their interactions, and I couldn't help but laugh.

Mom explained that before she knew him, Dad had been ordered into forced labor, along with most Hungarian men. They were used as mine fodder, preceding the German Army into Russia, to be blown up instead of the Germans. Dad escaped twice. The second time, he was taken to a camp and ordered to stand in front of a firing squad along with other escapees. Just before the shots rang out, the commandant decided to let the group go. It was his birthday, and he was in a good mood. Afterwards, Dad was moved to a camp in Austria, where he languished until the war's end. Apparently, the Nazis didn't want to waste more ammunition on Jews, hoping instead that they'd be infected with lice, and die of typhus or starvation.

My parents met after the war when Mom was in Budapest, selling items at an outdoor market. Dad asked her on a date, which she accepted only because she thought he was good looking and a Jew. She didn't care about finding happiness with a mate. In fact, Mom never hoped to find happiness for herself, because she had survived when most of her family had not. She suffered from survivor guilt all her life. All that mattered was getting married so that she'd have children to replace the family she'd lost.

When talking about, or to Dad, Mom was always demeaning. She described him as her third child. She claimed that, on their first date, Dad showed up at the door without flowers. She insisted that he leave and return with flowers, like a true gentleman. Dad did as she wished, and they were married soon thereafter.

I have their black and white wedding picture, which somehow endured. It, too, was bent, torn, and stained. I had it repaired, and it, too, hangs on my wall near Mom's childhood family picture. In it, Mom is wearing a borrowed black coat, which is all she had that was nice enough to wear. A small corsage is pinned to her coat. She and Dad are smiling sweetly at each other while several remaining family members, mostly Dad's, look on.

For almost four years they lived in a DP camp in Bamburg, Germany, awaiting sponsorship to the USA. My sister was born in that camp in 1946, and two years later, Mom was pregnant with me. My mother's Uncle Ben owned a summer resort in upstate New York called The White House. He and his family sponsored our family in exchange for work in the resort. Mom cooked for hundreds of guests, while Dad worked in the gardens. They were discouraged from talking about, or thinking about, their experiences during the war.

My Debut and Early Days

As the first American born member of my family, I was born in a Kingston, New York hospital on November 26, 1949 after my parents and sister traveled to Ellis Island literally with the clothes on their backs. They had been transported on a Navy ship, the USS Marlin Martin. After I was delivered, the doctor suggested naming me "Marilyn" after the ship.

We kids were left to ourselves at the summer resort, living and eating in the area reserved for "the help." One of my most searing memories from that time was that I caught a horrible case of poison ivy. To keep me from scratching the unbearable rashes all over my body, I was restrained by straps in the bed. I must have been about two years old when this happened.

When I was five, we moved to the Boyle Heights area in Los Angeles. Both of my parents worked hard, six days a week. Mom worked at two jobs, at night at Revell, an assembly plant making model kits for hobbyists, and during the day in a bakery in the predominantly Jewish Fairfax district. She wanted to be there for my sister and me as we were growing up. Dad worked as a gardener at Park LaBrea Towers. Between the two of them working, and not spending a penny on themselves or for non-essentials, they were soon able to purchase a small house in the Sunset Boulevard area. The other children in that neighborhood were all gentile, and it was in grammar school that I was first accused of "killing Christ."

When I was younger, I thought that being around Hungarian Holocaust survivors was normal. I glanced at, but thought nothing of, the tattooed numbers on their arms. While they danced joyfully to the czardas in our living room, their children and I hung out in the garage playing games.

Dad didn't participate in the living room socializing. He was a reclusive man, generally isolating himself in his bedroom after work. He insisted that dinner was at 6:00 pm, not a minute before or after. My sister and I pretty much ignored him. The only time Dad seemed visible was during the many explosive fights between him and my sister where I always acted as her figurative defense attorney. I just wanted him to go away since he had no clue about our family issues.

My role in the family became clear: I was to be the group therapist, trying to calm everyone's nerves and restore a semblance of order. I was ashamed to be associated with my family when I walked to school, hoping none of the neighbors recognized me. I was quiet and introverted, not wanting to draw any attention to myself or my family.

Dad's passion was classical music, which he listened to on a broken-down radio in his room. Although I generally tried to avoid having contact with my Dad, I took a high school music class in what I now realize was a feeble attempt to find commonality with him. As I walked down the hallway past his room, he'd see me, and beckon me to come in. He'd turn up the volume on a piece of music and challenge me to identify it. I'd say "Beethoven" or "Bach" or "Tchaikovsky," making sure that I was right. As much as it gave him pleasure that I knew the composer, he'd soon dismiss me from his room. It felt like a door had been slammed in my face, and it hurt – every time. I hated him, and promised to quit pandering to him, but I'd do it again and again, desperately wanting a relationship with my Daddy.

Dad was obsessed with his flowers, particularly the roses in front of our house. When neighborhood children playing ball accidentally stepped on one, Dad turned the hose on them. When friends came over to visit, Dad kicked them out precisely at 8 o'clock, his bedtime. He wasn't subtle about it. He shut off the lights and told them "go home." I was mortified. He became the neighborhood joke, something that further damaged my self-esteem.

I tried to keep our family dysfunction far from the eyes of others. My sister, who had arrived in America at age 3 and only knew Hungarian, was bullied in school for her inability to speak English correctly. She was emotionally ill and started seriously acting out. After barricading herself in her bedroom, she was hospitalized for several months in a mental institution.

I'll never forget how it felt when, on the drive home, my tearful mother asked me if she had done the right thing. I was 14 years old, angry, and only wanted to ignore this madness, put on a happy face at school, and pretend we were a normal family. In my subconscious attempt to prevent more sadness for Mom, I became the "perfect child" through high school. I got top marks in my classes, and kept any normal teenage angst internalized. During a counseling session between my mother and my sister, the social worker told Mom that it was I to whom they needed to pay attention. Mom mentioned this to me years later.

At 5'11" I was extremely tall, even while in grammar school. I suffered the indignity of playing the boy's part in May Day dances because there weren't enough boys. Towering over boys in my junior and senior high schools, I was never asked to dance or to go to proms and Grad Nights. I had exactly one date during high school where the boy, who I later learned was gay, didn't give me a goodnight kiss. That perceived snub made me feel even more different from my peers and added to my distorted beliefs about my femininity. It also didn't help that I was cursed by the agony of cystic acne, both during junior and senior high school. Even after dermatological treatments with my skin aflame, I would insist that Mom drop me off at school, cotton balls still attached to the bloody spots. No matter how ghastly I looked, I feared missing a test or an assignment.

I had a group of friends in my predominantly Jewish high school. Almost all the teenagers in my clique came from survivor families, although we never discussed it, nor did I know it at the time. My closest friend had a car, so we were able to go out for movies and pizza every weekend. When Mom insisted on slipping me $20 for the evening, I refused her money. My friends thought I was nuts, but how could I take the money when my mother spent nothing on herself?

Although no one in my family seemed to notice, I was horribly depressed. I tried to blend in with the walls of my high school, wishing I were invisible. Only in the academic sphere did I have some control over my life, as my achievements were recognized enough to bring my mother a measure of happiness.

I was unable to share my everyday problems with my parents. My focus was on them and how they were doing. One summer, I spent almost every waking moment with my face in a book. I took it to meals and shut out the world by staying in my room. No one noticed. I listened continuously to Simon and Garfunkle's song "I am a rock." It was my desire to become an emotional "rock," unable to feel anything, and to steel myself to the sadness and loneliness inside.

The Grown-Up Years

After college, I started to drink heavily. All the unspoken pain I had endured, along with my depression, transformed itself into rage. While I had been a quiet, nondescript young woman through my earlier years, I emerged as an angry drunk, anesthetizing my difficult experiences with drugs and alcohol. My parents never realized that I had a problem, even offering me extra wine at family dinners.

I didn't deal with feelings about the Holocaust until a fictional TV miniseries called "Holocaust" debuted in 1978. I was 29 years old. For the first time, a show dramatized a Jewish family's struggles to survive the horrors inflicted by the Nazis during World War II. Something snapped inside my head after one of the segments. I'd had enough of my parents' refusal to tell me about their war experiences. It had defined our lives, yet its impact was never discussed. I needed to know, and I was unwilling to wait any longer.

I drove to my parents' home, demanding that they tell me what had happened to them. Mom gave me a synopsis of what had happened to her and her family, but Dad's ordeal was not mentioned. I still wonder if he became the withdrawn man I knew because of the war, or if it was the effect of his earlier years.

I never "blamed" my father for my poor choices of men, but I'm pretty certain there were factors related to him that may have influenced my choices. It wasn't until college that I began to date. College boys in my commuter school seemed interested, but I found little in common with them. I was most attracted to non-Jewish boys, perhaps because I felt rejected by those in my high school.

When I was 18, I joined a volunteer group that tutored boys in Miller Probation Camp in the Malibu hills. Being around "delinquents" was new and exciting to me. I used my skills from being editor of my junior high and high school papers to start "Miller Highlights," a camp newspaper. A boy named Benny became the camp's first editor. He was just nine months shy of my age and had been incarcerated for selling drugs. He was cute and reminded me of a young Paul Newman in "Hud."

After graduating, he offered to return to the camp with me to help work on the newspaper. He lived in Van Nuys, so I picked him up by the side of the freeway on my way up the hill. As the relationship developed, I discovered myself becoming more and more attracted to him. He was quiet but interested in all facets of my life. He also played bass in a local rock band which only made him more appealing.

We couldn't have been more dissimilar. I was a Jew with European survivor parents. His family originally came from Oklahoma, lived in the Van Nuys barrio, and were observant Jehovah's Witnesses. Still, there was something comforting and familiar to him, and I began to experience romantic feelings.

Finally, he asked me out on a date to a Donovan concert at the Hollywood Bowl. I think he kissed me goodnight. We got married a few years later when I was 22. Even on my wedding day, I knew I was making a mistake. He was from another world, had dropped out of high school, and was unemployed. By the time we separated a year or so later, I was pregnant. When my son Shawn was three months old, I formally ended the marriage. I didn't know where Benny moved to and wanted neither support nor contact following the divorce.

Like many children of survivors, I hoped to begin a career in social work or another field where I could help "fix" others. After I graduated from college, jobs like that were unavailable. For a short time, I worked in an insurance company to make ends meet. When the company went bankrupt, I had no idea how to support myself and Shawn. Ironically, soon afterwards, I had my first interview as a deputy probation officer in Los Angeles County. The time I'd spent volunteering at Camp Miller came in useful.

During Shawn's early years, my drinking escalated. I dated random men, bringing many of them home. I knew I was an irresponsible mother and truly felt like scum, but I was very sick from alcohol and drugs. At age 30, I met my future husband, Wayne, at a country and western bar. Although I was into rock, not country, we met during the Urban Cowboy phase. We were both intoxicated, and I invited him home. As I wrote in a memoir called "Starting at Goodbye," I believed he'd be a one-night stand, but we stayed together, on and off, for almost 30 years.

Wayne's mother was a recovering alcoholic, so I learned a bit about AA (Alcoholics Anonymous) from literature she dropped off at our house for Wayne to read. Although I believed he was the alcoholic, at age 38, I realized my life was out of control. I went for help, and my therapist required me to attend AA meetings.

On January 4, 1988, I got sober and haven't had a drink since. When Wayne continued drinking, I ended our marriage. By then, we'd had a second child, Alanna, who was already four years old, named after Mom's murdered sister Ilona. Wayne and I shared custody, and I watched him get sicker and sicker. Finally, I invited him to an AA picnic to see sobriety could be fun. Six months later, he became sober and we remarried.

In those AA meetings, there were constant references to a "G-d of our own understanding." I didn't believe in G-d and felt this might jeopardize my sobriety. The Holocaust was my proof that if G-d existed, he wouldn't have allowed this to happen to my family and six million Jews.

I made an appointment with Arnold Rachlis, a Reconstructionist rabbi. Rabbi Rachlis, or "Arnie" as the congregation called him, asked about my family's formal religious experiences. When I was in elementary school, I had attended Sunday school in a Reform temple, but lost interest soon thereafter. I described our family's religion as "Holocaust Judaism."

Throughout her life, Mom was member of a synagogue, tending towards Orthodox ones. As a charming Holocaust survivor, she was a cherished member of any synagogue that she joined. Dad, on the other hand, was never religious. He only attended *shul* (synagogue) if Mom dragged him to a service. Our family celebrated major Jewish holidays together, during which Mom cooked the symbolic foods. We rapidly recited the blessings before eagerly moving on to eat her delicious cooking.

Arnie asked if I'd be willing to let Alanna experience Judaism as a joyful force in her life. I decided that I didn't want her growing up with my bitterness towards religion, wrote a check, and signed us up as new members that day. Although Wayne came from a religious Lutheran background, he was always supportive of Judaism.

Alanna attended religious school twice a week while studying for her Bat Mitzvah. I dedicated her custom-made prayer book to Ilona's memory. I knew that would deeply touch Mom. Alanna did a masterful job of leading a service in Hebrew.

I still hadn't dealt with my issues about the Shoah and antisemitism. This was made worse by the fact that Huntington Beach, where I lived, had become known as "The Skinhead Capital of the US" after a heinous hate crime. In response, on May 6, 1996, the Huntington Beach City Council unanimously adopted the Declaration of Policy about Human Dignity, which basically affirmed that hate would not be tolerated. This touched me deeply, so I sent a letter to two council members to thank them, while adding that my parents were Holocaust survivors.

Councilwoman Shirley Dettloff invited me to be a member of the newly created Task Force to monitor the situation in our city. I had never been a part of a city government entity before and accepted the offer with honor. Being on the Task Force changed my views. I realized that there would always be a small minority of haters who will never end their enmity towards those they view as the "other," although the majority is much more tolerant.

After leaving the Task Force, I continued being involved in community programs about the Holocaust. After a local educational television station announced the screening of a film on the lives of a survivor family, I invited Mom to come with me to see it. When the film's director asked if there were any survivors in the audience, my mother tentatively raised her hand. The moderator handed Mom a microphone to capture her comments. Until that time, she had never shared her story publicly.

It was as if a dam had burst. She began tearfully telling her story, making it difficult for the producers to cut her off. After all, the focus was to be on the family in the film. As I drove her home, Mom excitedly asked whether what she'd said was good. I assured her that she'd been wonderful. From then on, my mother accepted countless speaking engagements at Holocaust-related events. Once she got started, she couldn't stop, and was eventually interviewed by the Steven Spielberg Project. Her testimony, along with hundreds of other taped survivor testimonies, is preserved in the Washington DC Holocaust Museum. I'm so proud of her.

Enter "The Second Generation List"

Around 1999, I discovered a private, online, Second Generation group created by Paul Foldes, on the Shamash website. There, I first heard the term "memorial candle," the member of a family of survivors who was most involved in keeping the memories alive. I was my family's "memorial candle," and I now found others much like myself. Jumping in with both feet, I wrote prolifically and openly about previously suppressed feelings, describing nightmares of being pushed into a swimming pool brimming with gas. Others related to my Holocaust associations when I saw the word "showers" at a camping bathroom.

Not only did I feel safe talking about the effect of the Holocaust on my family and myself, but I also began to view many members as nonjudgmental friends with whom I could discuss everyday problems.

In December 2003, while I was on The List, Wayne was diagnosed with brain lymphoma. This nightmare was a major source of my posts. I needed as much support as I could find during this journey. Not only did the members understand and empathize with my frustrations, fears, and sadness, struggling to be his caregiver while working full time, but they also offered invaluable suggestions. Many of the members were going through, or had gone through, similar turmoil, so we were able to share each other's experiences, strength, and hope.

While I was at work, it was easy to "chat" by computer with the group, whose members came from different parts of the world. I got to know these people who were names on a screen about as well as my "real life" friends. Just as happens in most groups, I formed a raging resentment toward one List member that lasted for much of my first year. I shared personal details about my beliefs, while she had a different perspective and manner. This quarrel got ugly and contributed nothing of value to the group. I probably acted out my internalized family dynamics of arguments and anger on an easy target, a name on a screen.

She and I bumped heads early in the game. It became a power play, a challenge to find out which of the other members "sided with" whom. During this dispute, some members contacted her in private emails, while others did the same with me. I learned that this woman held a lot of influence in the religious Jewish community, and some feared antagonizing her.

I tried avoiding her, even deleting her posts unread. Still, there was a stubborn part of me that refused to be intimidated by her, and I occasionally read and responded to her online assertions.

This animosity was petty, destructive, and childish, causing much discomfort to the rest of The List. One member actually attempted to broker a truce via a three-way phone call. In it, my nemesis alleged that I needed to be the "center of attention." Maybe it was true. But she also alleged that I'd gotten the FBI to investigate her and her husband, a totally delusional claim. The truce ended unsuccessfully, each of us retreating into our own corners and continuing the battle.

I was sent a private admonishment by the then group administrator who accused me of involving the group in another "skirmish" between the two of us. Reacting impulsively, I immediately quit the group. Maintaining contact with the people I liked through private emails, I attempted to create my own unofficial List by sending "group" emails, hoping to keep up with the lives of people I'd come to cherish while avoiding my "enemy." How childish this game got to be, and how disturbing it was to everyone.

One wrote to me, "My heart sank when I saw the beginnings of the same drama unfolding. I know she drives you crazy, but can't you continue on The List (and getting the support of so many) while just ignoring her? Most of us can see and judge what's going on..."

When I got a long-distance call from Esther in Israel who urged me to return to The List while I sorted out the nightmare of my life, I realized how desperately I needed the help of its members. I couldn't do without the assistance of the individuals who cared and offered invaluable support while I forded one frightening development after another with Wayne and his cancer. I missed clarifying aloud in posts exactly how I was doing on a daily basis.

Having rejoined The List, I was welcomed back, feeling such relief as we reconnected again. Without having ever met me, these people knew me. They knew the members of my family and supported me through the difficulties I endured, just as I did with them and theirs. My involvement with the 2g (Second Generation) List allowed me to delve into buried emotions, particularly grief.

From the religious Jews on The List, I learned how Judaism deals with the death of loved ones in *shiva* services. I realized that I had never officially mourned the deaths of my family members murdered in Auschwitz. I announced to my immediate family that I was sponsoring a *shiva* service on the beach. I created a booklet of prayers and passed out copies to everyone with the ocean's crashing waves as a backdrop.

The service took an interesting turn when Mom and Ada shared recollections about their parents before the Holocaust. Until then, I knew very little. Mom described loving memories, especially of her father, occasionally looking to Ada for confirmation. Both sisters grew animated as the rest of us listened enthralled with the tales. What a nice change from all the sadness.

The following weekend, I invited them to my house so that I could videotape their recollections of these good times. After two hours interviewing Ada and Mom, I was about to conclude the tape. Suddenly, my father asked if I wanted him to tell his "story" on camera.

As he hesitantly spoke, Mom frequently interrupted him. I had to admonish her to let him talk. It was clear Dad's cognition was limited after having had brain surgery years before. Most surprising to me was that he was unable to articulate his feelings for his beloved Mom, no matter how I prompted him with questions about love. It was then that I had a huge realization. It wasn't that Dad didn't love me, but rather that he had no concept of its meaning. Much of the anger I'd always felt toward him lifted. He had no idea what love meant.

When Wayne lost his battle with cancer five years later, I turned to The List for support. They helped me deal with his death more intimately than did people close to me. I didn't have to explain the backstory. They had been there to hold my hand during those awful five years. On October 30, 2008, I wrote: "I am touched by the outpouring of concern and caring from this list, which has seen me through some of the worst and best times of my life." They shared memories of Wayne without having ever met him. I wrote, "Memories must, in fact, sustain me now, as they are all I have left of this loving, kind, and wonderful man with whom I shared twenty-eight years of my life."

We were people who'd only known death out of a more "normal" sequence, typically the deaths of grandparents, then parents, then those of our generation. Death had previously been an experience we'd known from afar, through the murders of our family members. I could laugh and cry with these people who understood grief as most cannot.

With the knowledge and support of The List, I retired from probation in 2005 and directed my sadness over Wayne's death into constructive action by helping veterans at the Long Beach VA nursing home. With the examples outlined by others on The List, I turned feelings of helplessness about animal cruelty into productive action by becoming a Humane Society district leader fighting for animal protection.

I met and married Mark in 2008. The relationship suffered from unresolved grief, and we divorced soon thereafter. We remarried, divorced, and remarried for the third time last year. Don't ask! People on The List never judged my decisions.

My two children are now adults, and each has his or her own children. My grandchildren are Colin, Owen, and Ava. I have expressed to The List that I don't revolve my life around being a Bubbe, but the happiness radiated by other List Bubbes has rubbed off on me.

Both of my parents died years ago. My dad was 90 and in an assisted living home. Again, I turned to The List for help as he neared the end. I was the last person to be with him while he lay semi-comatose and struggling for breath. I brought him a cassette of classical music pieces that I thought he'd enjoy. When I put on Hungarian music, his body writhed spastically. He hated Hungarians to the end. I switched to some Jewish melodies, which calmed him down, and gave him "permission" to go and to join his beloved mother.

Mom sank into progressive symptoms of dementia in her nineties. Her irrational paranoia resulted in her decision to move to Spokane to stay with Shawn. A year or so later, as her mind deteriorated, Mom agreed to return to California to live in a senior community near me. After picking her up from the airport, we stopped for a short meal at Dennys. Not 10 minutes later, while I drove home from the restaurant, Mom keeled over in the passenger seat. I screamed "What's wrong?", and she answered: "I don't know." Those were her last words. She was 97.

Retrospective on the Second Generation List

Over the years, The List has become an important presence in my life. Everything I've lived, I've shared with these people. The anger festering inside me during much of my life, which gave rise to that blow up with a List member, took years to dissipate. Perhaps I grew tired of the toll it took on my life. Anger is draining and is often aimed inappropriately. Eventually, my resentment towards that member ended, but not before it took a toll on the group. I'm not proud of my behavior, and hope I've made amends to the group over the years. Maybe that experience was what I needed to help me heal.

There were other times when I grew weary of The List's direction. When the main topic turned to illness and death of family members, I tried to steer people into other subjects. But just like my own experiences, this was what others needed to discuss.

I left The List a few times but always came back. No one had to beg me those times. It was the continuity and familiarity that made me return. I figured out my own issues, and was grateful to be allowed back in. Because of my religious family background, I had a push-pull difficulty with the subject. It was often those List members whose level of observance differed from my own, who compelled me to explore where I stand with Judaism. I am still unaffiliated, but my interest continues.

The List remained my own private outlet. While others in my immediate family knew I was involved, none was interested in joining the group, or hearing more about it. I have an observant Orthodox cousin in New York who visited Hungary, but I'm still primarily my family's memorial candle.

I formed many bonds that have endured almost 20 years, even meeting with some of The List members in real time. On an international trip in 2000, I arranged a stopover in New York City. Wayne and I were invited to stay in the home of Anita, a 2g who picked us up at the airport. When we met, it was as if we'd known each other forever. We reminisced about old memories without having to fill in the details. Several other New York members joined us.

We met Laurie when she came to California and met Mom. Wayne was still healthy then. Years later, when Wayne was in a wheelchair, we again met Laurie in Washington DC. Similarly, I met Sofia and her husband in New Jersey, and then again when they came out to California. I met Jake in Boston, and Esther and Evamk here in California. I still have on my office wall the mezuzah that Esther custom made.

Together, we mourned the deaths of our own. We learned about the untimely passing of List members Anne B and Colleen. Together, we pitched in to buy trees in Israel to memorialize them. We also shared our triumphs together. When Ruth got her PhD in Israel, we savored her accomplishment. When Judy B posted stories of her work in Holocaust research, we reveled in her achievements. Though we initially had disagreements, mostly about religion, I grew to love Judy and so many more of the more traditional members.

My life has been changed and helped beyond measure through my involvement in The List. I was able to clarify my thoughts and feelings, not only about my parents as survivors and about family murdered during the Shoah, but also how to deal with everyday struggles. I learned from where I got my strength, my resilience, and my passion for healing the world, from others who have shared a similar journey.

While I have not forgiven those who allowed the genocide of my people, much of the anger has healed. I still obsessively watch every movie and read every book I can about the Holocaust. That internal war will never end, but neither will my commitment to my parents and my family, NEVER to forget.

Dr. Paula David
The Outsider on the Inside

Introduction

When I first joined this Group, I suffered recurring bouts of Imposter Syndrome, and appropriately so. My parents were not Holocaust Survivors, but born in Toronto, Canada to Jewish immigrants who had left Eastern Europe in the early 1900s. My path to becoming a long-term active member of a group limited to adult children of survivors of the Holocaust, evolved from a series of happenstance. Decades ago, when I first joined, I sometimes felt like an intruder, a voyeur, or an imposter. Now this group is an integral part of my evolving sense of community, of friendship, of belonging and most of all, mutual caring.

As a young child, we lived with my maternal grandparents in a family-centric warm, boisterous, and loving household. I spent hours enveloped in my Bubbe's warm arms listening to her endearing Yiddish-driven stories of the Old Country. She talked about her life, but not so much about the people she lived it with, and often there was a dark inexplicable shadow hanging over her head. The noise behind those shadows was connected to any mention of the War and was made in hushed and secretive tones that became seductive to a child's ears. This cloud behind my Bubbe's smiling eyes was accompanied by distracted distressed looks when she would tell me of the family members whose names were now mine. My Yiddish name is Perele, named after her sister, murdered with her young family in the Holocaust. When my Bubbe called me Perele, she hugged even harder.

As I grew up, I learned more about the Holocaust, but references outside the confines of the family were few and far between. Ultimately, it was serendipity that introduced me to the world of Holocaust survivors and their families. When I met my husband, I understood that his parents were in Romania during the war, but by their own explanation, they were not Holocaust survivors. One had been sent to a labor camp, and one had been hidden by neighbors. Since they had not been deported to a death camp, they felt they were not "real" survivors. They rarely discussed their wartime experiences, nor did they recognize that their wartime trauma might impact how they subsequently lived their lives. My husband and I were both raised in Jewish homes, but shared little commonality within an experiential context of what that means. I attributed their differences to be familial, cultural, or influenced by recent immigration. I was so wrong.

This became apparent to me when I started working at a Jewish long-term care facility where over 70 % of the residents were Holocaust survivors. I was a trained social worker specializing in aging and found myself in a diverse community of older Jewish adults who had lived and experienced extreme trauma, changes, and challenges, not only beyond the expectations of my education but beyond my comprehension. When a unique opportunity arose, I took on the development of a new initiative within our facility as the Coordinator of the Holocaust Resource Project. My job was to develop a comprehensive and coordinated approach to understanding, educating, and caring for the specific needs of the relatively new population of aging Holocaust survivors and their families. I became immersed in a world of more questions than answers. It wasn't the knowing, but the not knowing that brought me to the Second Generation Group.

My Family; Knowing, Understanding and Feeling:

My parents were taught to feel fortunate for being born in a country that allowed them to live and grow up without pogroms, have access to education and health care, all while maintaining their Jewish identity. My maternal grandparents came from Brzeziny, Poland, and my father's mother's family immigrated with her family from Zhytomer, then part of the Russian Empire. My father's family came from Talne, not far from Zhytomer. That grandfather arrived on his own, eventually sending for some siblings and his mother. All these ancestors lived modest lives in the Old Country and suffered under oppressive and restrictive anti-Semitic regimes.

My mother's parents got married to flee Poland as a couple, and they arrived in Toronto with their forged passports, no money, exhausted, and four months pregnant with my mother. She was their "Blue Ribbon Canadian Baby" and the focus of her parents' hope, purpose, and sense of belonging in this strange world, far from home. The young couple moved into the heart of Toronto's Jewish immigrant community, living in a small three-bedroom home that also housed three additional young, struggling, newcomer families. Yiddish was the language of settlement in the heart of this neighborhood and my mother did not speak English or use her English name until she was registered in Kindergarten. Her mother was very excited to have a child in the school system and was looking forward to her little student passing on her new skills. A kindly Italian neighbor had been tutoring my Bubbe in English. She faithfully practiced and learned five new words per day. It wasn't until my five-year-old English-speaking mother had been in school for a few weeks that she discovered the language her mother had been learning and practicing was Italian. From that day on, my mother became the designated "Canadian Tutor" of the family!

My father was also born in Toronto. His parents were teenagers when they arrived, and they met after they had been living here for a few years. Their first child arrived almost immediately, and my grandmother was pregnant again a few years later. Sadly, my father's mother died within weeks of his and his twin sister's birth, and while neither of my parents had idyllic childhoods, my dad's was fraught with custody issues, blame, sadness and loss. His father remarried, had more children, and the reconstituted family also became "real" Canadians. That phrase, which I heard often, symbolized many layers of difference that I only recognized slowly over time.

In this new land filled with promise, both my parents experienced antisemitism in a city that had been predominantly white Anglo-Saxon Protestant, and was having difficulties adapting to the influx of Italian, Portuguese, Chinese, and Jewish immigrants in "their" Toronto. It was not always easy, and my mother would tell stories of her mother ensuring that her four children would become as Canadian as possible. When there wasn't enough money to properly feed everyone, my grandmother paid for my mother to take elocution classes to ensure she wouldn't speak like a *greener* (newcomer, immigrant). Pierced ears were *verboten* (forbidden), as was the sprinkling of Yiddishisms in English conversation. In my Bubbe's eyes, they were a sure sign of Old Country origins and therefore potentially dangerous. It seemed that the focus of all the parents of that time in that community was to raise their children to succeed and belong to this new world, while simultaneously to never take that belonging or succeeding for granted. Becoming a "real" Canadian was an ongoing theme; remaining a committed Jew was an assumed imperative. Both were an ongoing challenge.

Much as her parents were so proud to be Canadian, they also taught my mother to constantly look over her shoulder to ensure she wasn't the only Jewish child in a group. In school, the expectation was that my mother would be an overachiever, so that as a Jew, her right to attend would never be jeopardized. This deep-rooted insecurity and lack of trust in Canada's capacity or desire to accept Jews, seemed to hover in the air, and was an integral part of my mother's childhood. Intuitively, my mother ultimately passed that on to her children. My two sets of grandparents did not know each other until my parents began dating, but both families had similar views on their status and security in this county. Their children, my parents, were dating and getting to know each other when the War in Europe began escalating.

World War II was a very different experience for young Jewish adults living in Toronto than for those in Eastern Europe. Here, everyone knew war was approaching, and the men began to enlist voluntarily with the understanding there might be more choice and options regarding assignments and deployment. My mother and her sisters all married their boyfriends sooner than they planned, so that it was husbands they would be sending off to war rather than boyfriends. Once married, they returned to their parents' home as three young wives, while their men were deployed. My father enlisted in the Royal Canadian Air Force Officers Training Program. My mother and one sister both became pregnant in the early years of the war, before their new husbands were assigned to active duty. My older sister was born during that time and spent her first few years primarily being raised by the four waiting women at home.

My father once told me he left Toronto to go overseas as a patriotic young Canadian, expecting adventure while fighting for freedom. He had no idea that freedom barely touched the tip of the iceberg he was about to encounter. His overseas work was classified, and all his letters home were censored. Thus, the family in Toronto was left with only a multitude of silences blowing empty across the ocean. In the early days of the war, the few letters that were arriving from the many relatives still in the Old Country stopped abruptly. The silences grew more ominous in tandem with the rumors that ripped through the hearts of the Toronto Jewish community. Once the war ended and the rumors became the reality, the devastating losses impacted families differently.

There was an ironic dual and mixed reaction in Toronto from the Jewish community. My grandparent's generation was devasted as the extent of familial losses sunk in. They understood pogroms and anti-Semitism, but genocide was inconceivable. My parents' generation, mostly born in the New World, were left shaken, but also relieved when their men came back to pick up their lives again. When the men in my family returned home, my mother and her sisters became pregnant again, and not long after I was born, along with two cousins. I was born in an era of new post-war growth that was trying to take attention away from the atrocities that had occurred in Europe. While my family was beginning to look forward, the survivors were still trying to understand how and where to look at all. My parents remained in my grandparents' home, and the first few years of my life were spent wrapped in the love of two generations. We were one of the lucky families, our Canadian family was intact. However, as reports of the Holocaust became the stories of family losses back in Europe, the silences became louder, and there were no war stories in our home. Talk was of the potential of the future, and the past was quietly wrapped up and put away.

Finding Myself

When things get put away, they either tend to be forgotten or leave in their place a sense of absence or loss. I was never very sentimental about the past. As a teenager, I was focused on my future and defining my place in the world outside of the constraints, concerns, and consternation of my parents. I didn't even try to understand the layers of meaning and love behind my parents' plans and dreams insinuating on every aspect of my life. My mother was teeming with unfulfilled dreams and promise, deciding that only through her daughters would she find her fantasy of her perfect life. My father was infinitely more relaxed. As long as he could sit with his guitar or piano and sing to his girls, then all was right with the world. My parents' needs and wants were readily defined but inaccessible, and both were doomed to chronic frustration and elusive potential. Somewhere in my egocentric adolescence I did not notice or even care about those family desires, dreams, identities, and connections that had been put away.

It was the sixties and I wanted to be free, independent, self-determined, and just "go with the flow". The counterculture of the decade spoke to me, and I was determined to break loose of my perceived tethers to discover and embrace a new world defined by unilateral peace and inclusivity. I moved away from my parents' home and left suburbia forever. At the time, I interpreted my parents' silences, their insecurities, and their apparent overprotectiveness, as tethering my potential. In my search for this utopian love and peace, I created utter turmoil for myself. I dropped out of high school, found an alternative art school, spent hours over countless cups of coffee debating the meaning of everything, and wallowed in both my insights and my angst. I poured my heart into my art and created large canvases screaming with color and underlying confusion. I was part of a vibrant counterculture immersed in re-defining self-expression and the world. I joined my generation in singing about it, creating artwork about it, marching about it, and rallying about it, all in the name of justice and peace. It was a time of personal exploration, an emerging evolution of the women's rights movement, of protests against global and local inequities, and collective cries for change, all within a pulsating rhythm of power and hope. We were going to be the agents of change and had arrived just in time! The youth of the sixties felt that they had personally discovered both the tidal wave of social problems, and a shared vision of fixing them. It never occurred to me that my grandparents and my parents shared those feelings just as reverently, albeit in a different context and culture.

It was during this period that I met Lee; the man who would become my life partner and would join me in defining what was and would be important in our lives. At first glance, we were complete opposites, and in hindsight, the fact that we were able to quickly move past our obvious differences was significant. I was born in Canada, a high-school dropout, trying to move away from family expectations, trying to re-define my personal identity, raised in a safe and inclusive environment, surrounded by a large and loving family, and burdened with internal struggles and questions. He was born in Romania, the only child of Holocaust survivors from families that had been fractured and decimated by antisemitism, chronic loss, and the Holocaust. His childhood had been one of distracted struggling parents, oppression, a desperate need for relocation and immigration, learning new cultures, new languages, new countries, all within a family of three, under siege, and functioning on their own. Parental expectation and individual self-determination in his world were light years away from mine. His experience of family life, a child's sense of entitlement and security, were also light years away from mine.

When we met, he was a serious student both at the University and in life, having taken on his quest for knowledge and understanding on his own. His parents assumed nothing less. I had always navigated my path in a collective of some sort, while he embraced his personal and academic explorations individually. My parents were born into a world of promise and hope, his into a world of oppression and loss. Yet underneath our differences, we discovered our core values were much the same, the substance of our hopes for the future were the same, and our family tendencies to "put things away" and not talk about them, were also the same. We both came from a long history rich in tradition, hope, persecution, loss, and survival that was also the same. In those days, we were only thinking about being in love and how we would live our infinite tomorrows.

For the first time in my life, I felt I was acknowledged and loved just as I was, and that feeling allowed me to finally explore and embrace new challenges and directions. I began to feel like a bona-fide "Real Canadian". We married, moved to another city, ostensibly to attend school, but mainly to attend to creating our new family of two, and begin to build a life together.

I joined him at the University, and we spent the next few years learning and beginning to integrate our different pasts and potential future. Together we embarked on new learning curves. We were aware of the academic ones, but less so of the familial ones.

In the final year of completing our graduate degrees, we welcomed our first child. We also decided to move to a rural area and begin the next chapter close to family, but with space to define and develop ourselves independently. It was a good choice, and it was there that we both began our respective careers, settled into an inclusive and new lifestyle, and grew our own nuclear family. We had arrived in this small town with one baby and two freshly minted degrees and left with five children, a wealth of work experiences in our respective fields, a wide variety of new opportunities taken, a host of strong friendships, community involvement, and family adventures. Living in a rural community offered us choices and opportunities that we would never have experienced in a large city.

After over a decade of living and loving our new lives, much to the confusion of our children, Lee and I decided to move back to the city. We made this difficult choice to enable our children to explore the many and diverse educational, recreational, and social choices available. Most of all, we wanted them to have easy access to the unconditional love of their grandparents and extended family. We had learned to understand and appreciate the critical role of tradition, history, identity, and acceptance that family can provide. For me, it took a dramatic move to rural Ontario, surrounded by families who had worked the land for generations, took care of themselves and each other, and enjoyed living in a community that sustained and nurtured them. We wanted our children to feel this within the context of their own relatives and their family history.

We had been the only Jewish family town, and while it made our children feel special, it also contributed to their limited understanding of what that meant. The move was much more about people than place. It wasn't an easy transition for any of us, and I often considered and reconsidered our circumstances, compared to those of Lee's parents and my grandparents when they were making their way to Canada. I developed a whole new appreciation and gratitude for their choices, their courage, and their capacity to adjust and readjust when they relocated and turned their lives upside down. First, they adapted. Then, they thrived. Although on a very different scale in a very different time for very different reasons, when we packed up and moved our family, we did the same.

Discovering The List

Once back in the city, we established our new home, settled the kids into their new schools, and Lee and I made some major career moves as we started our new jobs. After years of working in child welfare, in 1988, I began my journey into the world of older adults and the practice of Gerontology. I was hired as a social worker in a renowned Jewish long-term-care multi-service facility. Within a month of starting at Baycrest, I knew I had found my place. I brought a lot of diverse experience to the position, was a seasoned social worker, but ultimately, completely unaware of the rewards, the adventures, the learning, and the satisfaction waiting for me. I had always associated aging with illness, loss, and death. I had no idea that within those landmarks and major events lay so many life stories, each one richly interfaced with the fabric of my own identity, family, religion, culture, city, country, and history.

Baycrest's continuum of care services include a long-term care facility, supportive housing, a community center, independent living accommodation, an older adult hospital and a multitude of community clinics, professional healthcare services. The majority of patients, clients, and consumers are Jewish, and my tenure at Baycrest coincided with the beginning of the major cohort of Holocaust Survivors reaching out for age-related healthcare. At that time, we were unaware of the unique needs and services that they might require as they navigated the range of age-related challenges. Not only was I new to a gerontology focus; I was also new to working with survivors and their families and the impact of severe trauma and loss.

I quickly learned that within my client base, the families of many Holocaust Survivors questioned our services. Often, my work for this population required more support than other identified groups. I decided to invite the adult children of my clients who were survivors to a group meeting and ask them how and what supports we might adapt, to better accommodate their needs. I wasn't sure if the evening was going to be an information exchange, an educational event, the beginning of a mutual aid group, or just an opportunity to vent at the social worker. It turned out to be all of these, and the beginning of a remarkable adventure for everyone involved. That group eventually became the core of a community-based 2nd Generation Group that is still in existence today, over 30 years later! From our original meeting, we also recognized the need and potential for a survivors' group and eventually had two; one for residents, and one for community members. As the years went on, and the aging Child Survivors began using our services, we started a group specifically for Child Survivors. We learned and grew together, and all four groups thrived.

These groups were also the beginning of my education and evolution of understanding of the range of unique challenges of survivor families. At the time, the key experts in the field were primarily the survivors and their children, and the existing literature was slowly evolving and expanding. A specific focus on older survivors and age-related challenges had barely begun, and the possibilities of evidence-based practice were in the very early stages.

As well as being a challenging and rewarding work experience, much of what I learned from these various groups informed and enriched my personal life. I developed a new perspective on my in-laws, and new insights into the many traumatic events they had survived but chose to never discuss. I began to understand themes of over-protectiveness, poor boundaries, and a deep-rooted restlessness. I began to understand what my husband had missed, and the toll that growing up without a supportive network or extended family takes. I began to understand the conflictual combinations that survivors and their families faced, including deep seated disappointment and expectation, relief and concern, pride and shame, and feeling totally insecure within a new-found security. I hadn't realized that these feeling were part of many common denominators within survivor families, and how they directly impacted me and my family. It was both exciting and discomfiting to be on the edge of so much new learning. When I discussed this with my husband, he was unsure. He had been raised by parents who denied being survivors of the Holocaust, so he did not feel the sense of commonality that I was just beginning to appreciate. At that time, he did not identify as member of the "Second Generation".

As I navigated my way through a new chapter in my work and in my household, I was continuously looking for new resources and knowledge. Within our Group, one member kept referring to his "other" Second Generation Group; what those members thought about a certain topic, how they voiced their opinions, what problems they dealt with etc. I was intrigued. I really thought we were the first and only mutual aid group in the city for adult children of survivors and was excited to hear we might discover new resources and experiences. It turns out his other group was an online moderated one, the members scattered around the world, and was only open to children of survivors. I reached out, introduced myself, and asked if I could join. I wanted to learn and understand to better support my Group.

At that time, Jake and Paul were the moderators on the online Second Generation Group. Jake sent me a prompt and polite rejection. This was a "family based" group, not for professionals, and restricted to adult children of survivors. I wrote back and explained part of my quest for understanding and my interest was rooted in my need to better understand my own family. My children were 3rd generation, my husband was 2nd generation, and his parents claimed they weren't "real" Survivors of the Holocaust. I explained that I was recognizing similar patterns in the lives of the Holocaust survivors at work. as those within my own family. I realized I had a great personal knowledge gap and lack of understanding, and I wanted help in understanding and being part of a survivor family. Jake took my request to the Group, and they voted to let me join. I remember the ironic satisfaction I felt with the acceptance of the Group!

In those early days, new members gave detailed self-introductions, usually describing their parents Holocaust experiences, countries of origin, current life circumstances, and some basic challenges existing within their personal stories. I was totally intimidated by both the complexities of lives described, and how my story was so deeply different. My parents had never stood in the face of torture, death, and global insanity. My parents were not ripped from their lives, their families, their homes, and the people they loved. My parents, by elimination, were "normal". I guess others had similar reaction, because the immediate response to my presence was lukewarm, and I was on the Group's site reading far more than writing and interacting.

Once I became a more active participant, I discovered another aspect of my "difference". My awkwardness, my reticence, and my silence were not in reaction to hearing their personal family stories, but by being labelled as "not Second Generation, but normal". Conversations would take place where someone would describe dysfunctional behaviors or approaches to child rearing by their parents, and other would chime in with total understanding. Often, someone would turn to me and ask me if indeed that particular incident was "normal". Even while cyber-chuckling in response, I was burdened by a deep dark secret and didn't know how to share it... I was nowhere near "normal". Slowly over time, we came out of our protective shells, shared more openly and more inclusively. We learned how to listen through a keyboard and see each other with our inner eyes. The List did evolve into a strong ongoing conversation that fostered an equally strong community, but it was not for everybody.

Membership in a Listserve like ours is based on self-selection that is predetermined by some common traits. When our List began, this type of virtual relationship was still fairly new, and we found ourselves exploring both the issues at hand, as well as the evolving use of the technology. In those days, not everyone had a computer, which excluded an unknown potential. Once connected, we had to be adept at typing/keyboarding to be able to jump in and write out our thoughts, experiences, and points of view. Those who couldn't easily express themselves through the written word, didn't last. By self-selected functional elimination we ended up with an articulate, expressive, and opinionated group of people, who enjoyed the role of narrative in their written communications.

For many of us, regardless of theme, it was a first opportunity to be part of an interactive, ongoing dialogue with people scattered around the world. At times, amid a heated discussion, I would have to go to sleep at night, and let the other hemispheres continue the conversation. Before I left for work in the morning, I would go online to check what the Israeli contingent thought about the current topic. I'd check to see if the Australians had caught up with the newest input. I grew to appreciate and respect the diverse range of opinions, and the ensuing debates over so many topics.

As time went on, we continued to peel away more and more layers of protective shells and learn to trust the evolving intimacy. I realized then and still appreciate the choice the group made when it accepted me, and I never took my membership for granted. Perhaps, because I did not share the one major commonality that existed for the others, I sought out different common interests and experiences. It was my voice that often piped up to remind people that the issue under discussion was a common one, and not unique to the world of survivors.

Regardless of topic, within the dynamic of the relationships that developed, there was a core of people who bonded and shared openly. Overtime we grew close enough to trust each other with enough distance to maintain a sense of privacy and protection from our own disclosures. The virtual friendships supported a sense of safety, and the ongoing discovery of shared perspectives allowed true friendship to grow. Within the group of "regulars", some of us were fortunate to find one or more kindred spirits, and occasionally these friendships grew differently, some taken off list, and while still virtual, into a 1:1 dimension. Still, most of the conversations, whether reflective, philosophical, heated or occasionally mundane, were discussed within the complete group. Much to my surprise and pleasure, a group of people whom I had never even laid eyes on, became an important component and presence in my life.

Over time, any group that sustains intimacy, sharing, and caring will hit some roadblocks that will challenge the sense of well-being of its members. Our Second Generation Group seemed to do so on a regular basis. The nature of our virtual connections often developed into heated arguments which sometimes deteriorated into hurtful and dysfunctional online communication. These issues would cause great stress and upset, both for the moderators and the people directly involved. Reconciliation was never easy. Still, the virtual world allows a person to turn off their computer, walk away and return to the "real" world. At different times, over different issues, most of us pulled back and temporarily abandoned the Group.

That exit strategy was used sometimes because of hurt feelings that were difficult to work through online, sometimes just for a break from the intensity, sometimes to soothe hurt feelings, and sometimes just to back away for a bit and reflect. Occasionally, someone would erupt and manage to use the written word to effectively express fury, shouting, annoyance, and sometimes even insults. Pending the participants on a particular thread it could get volatile. With my personal difficulties with confrontation and yelling, I would get very uncomfortable. I learned to either shut down and retreat to the familiar silences of avoidance from my childhood, or jump in and stand behind my opinion. Easing into a standard of more mature communication in cyberspace allowed me to do better in the "real" world. It wasn't always easy, but always there was the undercurrent of new learning, new insights, and recognizing we were all filling in some challenging blanks within our own understanding of family and group dynamics. We realized we were often modelling our own family behaviors and norms on The List; for better or worse. The downside of this was that we had some hard and alienating arguments; the upside was that we strengthened our bonds and comfort level and extended our circle of trust and shared vulnerabilities.

For years we spent hours of time discussing our families, our relationships within those families, our thoughts on how our families of origin impacted our world views and our well-being, and how the Holocaust likely changed the trajectories of all these topics. Over the years, my sense of personal family expanded to include my in-laws, and I felt their presence as "my family". At some point, their issues, concerns, and relationships within my life became very relevant within the ongoing explorations of the Group. Within our Group we experienced divorces, new marriages, children leaving home to begin independent lives, and a host of topics that occur within families. I recognized that my children were also part of a survivor family, and through their father and their grandparents, they would have to learn and appreciate the complex feelings and responses to that experience and label. I realized that this Group that was always sitting quietly, waiting for me in a nook between my kitchen and TV room, was having an impact on me well beyond the notion of work resources. These people had become my friends, and a form of surrogate alternate family.

Sadly, with that level of attachment and involvement, we also experienced the hard parts of that bond. After several years of being together, we began to deal with a few premature deaths within our membership. That's when our physical distance impacted me personally, and I found these losses harder to deal with in an online environment. A particular challenging loss for me was the unexpected death of Shari. We had grown close and visited each other's homes; mine in Canada, hers in Israel. We corresponded regularly on and off The List. Losing Shari and sharing that with the Group was extremely important to me. The Group was able to sustain and process the discussions of loss, grief, and irreversible change. The dichotomy of our "far-away closeness" expedited these difficult conversations.

It wasn't always heavy and intense. We celebrated family milestones; Bar/Bat Mitzvot, birthdays, weddings, graduations and truly took great pleasure in each other's happiness. *Mazal Tovs*, good cheer, photos and details would fly around the time zones, and put very real smiles on the faces of our virtual friends. When my son, who has Down Syndrome, had his Bar Mitzvah at the age of 21, I shared his unique story with The List. The service was held at his Camp, was totally non-traditional and for his family... very special. The List response was typical and touching. Within minutes of posting, I received joyful *Mazal Tovs* from around the world, from List members who were secular, Orthodox, and every type of Jewish observance in between. People told stories of unusual Bar Mitzvahs in their own families, of family members with a range of different physical and/or cognitive challenges, and how they and their relatives dealt with those. Most of all, the Group shared its collective pleasure in my family's pleasure! I could tangibly feel the support and sense of shared excitement that I hadn't thought possible in an online environment.

As the years marched on, our discussions and updates matched our own maturing and developing. After a long-time focus on children and child rearing, we started sharing the worries and fears for aging parents, their illnesses, their challenges, and eventually their deaths. The death of a parent has a major impact on any adult child, and in a survivor's family there are often many added layers. The most obvious difference is the usual absence of a large family gathered around sharing the grief, the memories, and the strengths. Our Group was able to provide that in a very virtual way, giving new meaning and insight into the growing number of "online support groups". We had become a "family" of sorts, and our sense of that connection often mirrored both the benefits and challenges that are inherent in families. So many of our Group members did not have extended family and did not have the experience of sharing their lives with cousins, aunts, and uncles. Group members often filled in as surrogate "cousins" and were ready to stand by and be supportive. Over time, discussions were less about the Holocaust, and more about relationships, personal changes, evolving narratives, and the ability to know that we were surrounded within a safe and caring cyberspace.

Thirty Years Later: The List in My Life

Three decades of ongoing explanations and discussions of the inner, outer, perceived, and actual lives of a group of adults and their families would provide any explorer with a wealth of experience and memories. We have come a long way, literally and figuratively, and The List has accompanied us and remained relevant throughout. Today, the Second Generation List has evolved far from its origins, and only the fact of being part of a survivor family remains the constant. Most of the survivor parents have died, and List members themselves are now the Bubbes and Zaidas of their families. We celebrate new generations of children and grandchildren, and we celebrate that they will know aunts, uncles and cousins as they grow up. We celebrate our presence within this circle of growth and renewal. In fact, we celebrate anything we can within our membership, and we are quick to share our happiness with the Group whenever it occurs.

We are now the Family Elders and we recognize the responsibilities of ensuring that future generations will both honor the memories of their survivor great-grandparents, and understand how to move forward in strength and security. Many of us have learned to be better communicators around the hard topics and acknowledge pain and shortcomings in order to heal. We have learned to cherish whatever happiness, family accomplishment, or new joy that enters our Group. One of my greatest pleasures throughout my List life was following through on opportunities that occurred over the years for several of us to meet "in real life". To have a genuine bond of shared history and familiarity with a List member in a two-dimensional world, and then enter their three-dimensional world and see, hear, touch, and talk face-to-face, is a remarkable experience. I have met members of the Group individually and in small gatherings in London, Oxford, New York, Philadelphia, Florida, Haifa, Jerusalem, Tel Aviv, Toronto and Montreal, Ireland and Australia. We have travelled together, met each other's families, spent extended time together, gathered in coffee shops, restaurants and living rooms, attended conferences together, and most of all, laughed, and cried, and talked to each other...in "real life". Even though we have never all been in the same place at the same time, our random and varied small group meetings were important to all of us. We realized what a diverse group we still are, with different types of jobs, different family constellations, different nationalities, different political and religious beliefs, and different lifestyles. So different, yet we share a unique common bond; we are all members of the Second Generation Group, where through the potential of cyber communication, our core members have stuck together throughout, and we all care for each other.

Patrice Flesch
The Lie

Introduction

I grew up not knowing who I was. Our family history, as told to me, was all lies.

Our family lived in an antisemitic suburb of Manhattan. I was extremely ignorant about Judaism, and rarely came in contact with Jews. Or perhaps I did but didn't know it, because I was unfamiliar with what names were Jewish. I never even saw a bagel!

As a child, the only thing that interested me in Jewish versus Christian was Hanukkah versus Christmas. Was it better to get presents for eight nights or get one pile on Christmas morning?

I was sent to Sunday School, something I had no interest in. Our minister was Ralph Waite who later became a Broadway star, and eventually featured in a famous television show, The Waltons. But I was quite indifferent to what I was supposed to be learning and the only thing I enjoyed was Palm Sunday. Were all given palm fronds and proceeded to whack each other with them. As for Jesus, I didn't know who he really was, and didn't care. I attended Sunday school (not my choice) until I was 16 and managed to retain nothing.

After high school I went to college in upstate New York. Interestingly, almost all my best friends were Jewish. I didn't seek them out, it just happened naturally. They were all secular Jews, so I didn't learn from them about the Jewish religion, but rather about their food, customs, and culture. It was also the first time I had Black friends. Clearly, I had been very sheltered in my WASP neighborhood.

Spending most of my time with Jews made me wonder about my relationship to Judaism. I had known about the Holocaust at a very early age, but don't remember how I knew. My intuition told me that the Holocaust had something to do with me, and as my suspicions grew, I wanted to know more.

I chose a very inappropriate time to ask about my heritage. We were in Virginia visiting my sister. It was Easter Sunday, and we were at a restaurant having Easter dinner. I don't know what possessed me to do this at that time, but I blurted out "Are we Jewish?" My father's response was

"What does it matter?" Hmmm....Then he announced that his back hurt because the chair was uncomfortable and walked to another section of the restaurant.

Eventually, a waiter came to our table and told us that we needed to go to the other part of the restaurant to help my father. The three of us made our way over. My father was lying on the floor screaming, supposedly from his (non-existent) back pain. He made a big scene, and everyone in the restaurant was watching. I knew it was a diversion from my question. We finally got him up and out of the restaurant and I remember thinking: "Now I KNOW."

I always knew that my father was German. Even at a young age, I knew a lot about World War II. I just assumed that my father left Germany to get away from the war. There was nobody I could talk to because I had no relatives. My grandfather lived in Spain and I was aware that I had an aunt, uncle, and cousins in Colombia, but people didn't fly around so much in those days. So, the distance was a plausible reason for not meeting them and it seemed logical that I wouldn't have met these far away people. Curiously, I knew of an aunt, uncle, and cousins who lived a few hours away in Philadelphia, but my father said they kept to themselves, didn't have friends, and weren't particularly interested in knowing us.

The Proof

Although I felt rather confident that my father was Jewish, it took me about 30 years to begin researching his story.

The Flesch family was very prominent and wealthy. They lived in a luxurious house. My father had a nanny and went to the finest schools. He was the oldest of three children and had a younger brother and a sister. Despite his being a poorly behaved "problem child", he was his mother's favorite.

It was my Grandfather Herbert, a factory owner and CEO, who realized early on that Jews were headed for big trouble in Germany. Although it was against the law, he sent money and machinery to Brussels and Paris to start new factories. For these actions, he was arrested by the Gestapo and put in jail in 1934. That same year my father left his school, despite the fact that Jews had not yet been expelled from German schools. He made his way to Amsterdam where he fell in love with a substantially older woman, but his mother put an end to it.

In 1936, the Nazis made a proposal to my great-grandfather, the Chairman of the Board of the factories. He had to make a choice. His son Herbert would be set free if he signed the factories over to the Nazis. If not, his son would be sent to a concentration camp. My grandfather was set free, and the factories were signed over to the Nazis. Not trusting the Nazis to not send him to a concentration camp anyway, my grandfather immediately fled. With him was Patzi the nanny/secretary (who later became his 3rd wife), his sister and husband Max and Minnie (Flesch) Rothschild, and their son Wilhelm. They went to Brussels and Paris to pick up the money my grandfather Herbert sent there. Unfortunately, the Rothschilds remained in Paris where they were later arrested and sent to Auschwitz. They were all murdered.

Once Herbert and Patzi made it to Spain, Gerhart (my father's brother) joined them. The three of them took a boat to Baranquilla, Colombia where they started another factory and became wealthy again. My father's sister Inge later joined them. Her mother smuggled her out of rankfurt during Kristallnacht, bribing someone to make sure Inge's compartment wasn't opened. Other Jews were thrown off the train. So now, at the age of 15, Inge arrived in LeHavre and took a boat to Colombia. She remembers eating a lot of food at the gate. Wearing an eyelet dress when she arrived, her father, who constantly undermined her confidence, told her that she looked like a big fat swiss cheese.

My father Peter had a sponsor in the United States, and in 1938, he took a ship from Rotterdam to Hoboken, N.J. Upon arrival, he dropped his middle name (Joachim) and changed his birth date so that he would be difficult to trace. Once in New York, he began his life as a Christian, certainly not a Jew.

His mother Hilde eventually left her second husband to be with my father in New York. There she was reunited with her best friend and lover, Hannah Arendt. Her friends were an intellectual, artsy group. Hilde also had a romantic relationship with Paul Tillich. Unfortunately, Hilde died of breast cancer soon after arriving.

My father began his search for a WASP wife and went to social events at the Riverside Church. There he found his perfect wife, my mother Ethel Sulkins. Ethel was the oldest of three sisters. Her sister Edna died as a teenager from kidney disease, but the third sister, Annette, is still alive at the age of 102!

My parents started dating, but by summertime Ethel was at her family's beach house. This posed a problem for my father because, since he was a German (and an alien), and it was wartime, he was confined to a small geographic area. His solution was to change his address every Friday and Monday so he could visit. Eventually, immigration caught up with him, and he was permitted to visit his fiancé at her summer home.

My father married into the Sulkins family, people of Irish and German heritage. Ethel's father was a very adventurous daredevil and lots of fun. He was the fifth person in Massachusetts to obtain a driver's license. He would drive to Florida in one go at 100 miles an hour and outdrive the police who chased him. One of his greatest achievements was stealing a piece of Plymouth Rock! Her mother Liberty was named after the Statue of Liberty. My mother Ethel was the prim and proper type as opposed to her sister Annette, who was the more outgoing adventurous type. When my parents got married, they spent a lot of time with Annette and her husband Gardner.

Then I was born, not knowing that I was embarking on a life full of lies.

What a Strange Life

I arrived in the world on June 23, 1951, the same day my family was moving from Manhattan to Long Island. Already I was trouble. While my mother was giving birth to me, my father was inefficiently overseeing the move.

The number 23 played a significant role our family's lives. When our family moved the second time, the final move, it was on the 23rd, my eighth birthday. I graduated from high school on the 23rd, 1969. My father escaped from Europe on the 23rd and married my mother on the 23rd.

The first move was to a middle-class immigrant neighborhood. The second move was to a wealthy, antisemitic town. What a perfect cover for my father! How could he be Jewish and want to live there?

I was forced to attend a Christian church, something I had no interest in. At school I was bullied for being the tallest girl in the class. At home, my father was constantly screaming. Yet to the outside world, he was affable and charming. I was attacked on both fronts, school, and home.

I was the bad child, and my older sister was the good child. She was able to be the good child because she was in denial, never seeing what was actually going on right before her eyes. She continued this denial throughout her entire life. Her husband left her to live on another continent after two years of marriage. She behaved as if she still had a husband, and the rest of us played along. I was the normal one, reacting to the lunacy of my family. But that made me bad, and my parents sure did a good job of making their feelings known to me.

Happy to leave my home, I went off to college where most of my friends were Jewish. I was unaware of this for a long time. I had been so sheltered, that I didn't even know what a Jewish name was. I just seemed to gravitate towards them. I finally had a bagel and Chinese food!

I spent one year of college in London, going to school and working as a barmaid. What fun! It was the best year of my life up until then. I believe that's where my love of travel began. To date I have been to 50 countries.

After graduating college, I went to photography school in Boston. The same thing happened there again, where I had mostly Jewish friends. Eventually, I married a Jewish man and I told him what little I knew about my family background. It didn't matter to him whether I was Jewish or not, yet I wonder whether that was a factor in my attraction to him. The irony is that I married a Jew, and my sister married an Austrian Nazi whose father had been in the Nazi party. My sister's husband was very racist. During Christian holidays, for the sake of my mother, I forced myself to go. It was a nightmare. To say that her family was very badly behaved is an understatement.

One example: My husband stated that on Christmas, his family went out for Chinese food. Franz asked: "Is that because Jews are so cheap?" This was typical of him. Pete and I would breathe a sigh of relief when Nicky's (my sister) family left.

My husband Peter was perfect. It was like I had married myself! We always had the same feelings and opinions. We never had to compromise because we both wanted the same things. Life with Pete was wonderful for about 20 years. He had my adventurous spirit, and we constantly explored the world. We both shared a love of dogs, and they became members of our family. We never had an interest in having children as there were too many other experiences that we wanted to have.

I was so lucky to have two careers that I loved. I had an exciting freelance photography business for about 30 years. The people I met, and the experiences I had, were invaluable. My work was more fun than my social life! When photographing celebrities, I took Pete along. I also photographed for non-profit causes that I loved. It was very meaningful to me to be able to help these causes through my photography. After about 30 years, I decided that I need to cut back on photography and add something else to my life.

Yoga was ma passion and I had been doing it for 25 years, long before it became a craze. I therefore got my teacher training certification and started a yoga business, eventually opening my own studio. I did fun things, like a fundraiser for the Animal Rescue League or holding a DOGA class, where people could do yoga with their dogs. It was very rewarding. I was told by many students that I had taken them out of pain, something their doctors had been unable to do. I made people feel better about themselves. Some students even said it was their substitute for going to church.

At this point, my life was going well. I had a great husband, two wonderful careers, traveled a lot, had many friends, and always had at least one dog about whom I was crazy. All of that changed when I got a phone call telling me that my mother had died.

After receiving the news, I immediately drove to New York. Even before I arrived, my mother's body was cremated. Nobody considered that I would like to have seen her. Then I found out the plans for the horrific "funeral" which my father arranged quickly and secretly. To dispose of her ashes at sea, he rented a tourist boat that gave tours about seals. My mother would not have wanted her ashes to be thrown into the ocean on a freezing cold day. I was not permitted to invite anyone to comfort me, and even my mother's sister and friends weren't invited. My father invited one of his friends, an obnoxious lawyer who was later sent to jail, me, my sister, and her two spoiled brat children.

As a photographer, I photograph everything that happens in my life. As my father was emptying my mother's ashes into the ocean, one niece screamed at me to stop taking pictures. Already hating her, I felt like throwing her overboard and listening to her scream as the sharks ate her. This was truly the funeral from hell. I wish I had never gone.

Because this was not a proper funeral for my mother, I decided that, out of respect for her, her friends, her side of the family and myself, I needed to have a second funeral. My Aunt Inge (my father's sister who he kept away from me) wanted to come to the funeral, driven by her son Steven. My father went berserk and said that they would be thrown out if they came.

My sister asked me why I thought he was behaving in this manner. I told her that it was because he didn't want his Jewish relatives in our church. She discounted my explanation, denying that our family was Jewish. Years later, I found out that when she was a teenager, she visited my grandfather in Spain and he had told her the entire story of our family and our Holocaust history. She conveniently forgot.

Before the second funeral, I wrote to my offensive niece Kim. I told her how I felt about how she had acted previously and told her to behave better at the second funeral. Instead, she teamed up with my other niece Courtney, and tortured me during the funeral. Afterwards, neither my sister nor father did anything about it.

After I returned to Boston, I had a nervous breakdown. The combination of my mother's death and my family's cruel behavior was too much to take. Again, none of them cared. From their response, I'm sure my nieces were quite pleased with the damage they had inflicted upon me.

Seriously damaged and broken, I sought out a psychiatrist whose parents were Holocaust survivors. He was helpful, but it wasn't enough. I wanted to talk to other children of Holocaust survivors. The internet was quite new, and I did a search and found that there was an email group that met my criteria. Technically, I'm not Jewish, I call myself a "Holocaust Jew", and I wasn't sure whether I would be accepted. Ruth Tenenholtz was the gatekeeper and she let me in. I was now a member of The List.

My Life on The List Begins

After my family's horrific behavior at my mother's funeral, I had less contact with them, and now, no contact at all. The List was to become my family for the rest of my life. Initially, it was very awkward. After all, I wasn't really a Jew like everyone else in the group. They used words I didn't understand. They seemed to know each other so well, and I didn't know anyone there. There were some Orthodox members, something I knew nothing about. As this often happened to me throughout my life, I felt like an outsider. It took a long time for me to be comfortable. Eventually, I sought their advice on various dilemmas. This group is very intelligent and very good at finding resolutions to problems.

I decided to track down the cousin who tried to drive my father's sister to the funeral, and because he owned a business, I was able to find him through a Google search. I wrote to him, asked him if he wanted to talk about personal things, and he immediately answered yes. Within minutes I was on the phone with him, asking why our family had left Germany. He laughed nervously and said it was because they were Jewish. I was so relieved to hear those words, confirming what I already knew.

Soon after, I met my aunt Inge and my cousin Steven (the two who had been denied entry to my mother's funeral) at my grandmother's (non-Jewish) cemetery in New York. This was the beginning of a close relationship with Inge and my two cousins. My aunt Inge had guessed that the reason for our lack of meeting was that my father was hiding our family's Jewish and Holocaust history. She was, of course, correct.

Next, Inge and I flew off to Baranquilla, Colombia where I met my aunt Rosita, uncle Gerhardt (my father's brother), and my cousin Herbert. Inge and I grew very close. It's like we were the same person. She said her mother was like us too. When she died, I was more upset than when my mother or father died.

It was interesting to hear my aunt and uncle talk about my father who had been a problem child, always getting kicked out of school, yet he was their mother's favorite. I had attributed much of his screaming to his experience with the Holocaust. Hearing that he had such behavioral issues, I wondered if the Holocaust was even connected to do with his current-day behavior. The group of us really bonded during that trip.

Another cousin, Eric, was supposed to meet me in Baranquilla, but asked me to come to Bogota. I did not have the clothes for that drastic temperature change, and I searched to no avail at a shopping mall for clothes for someone of my height. Finally, a tall family friend provided me with her wardrobe which fit perfectly, so off I went to Bogota. I enjoyed my visit with Eric, his wife, and kids. Since Eric worked, he hired a chauffeur to drive me around so I could see Bogata. Quickly, I realized that my cousin's intent was to keep me indoors. Being a photographer, I wanted to walk around and take photos. The chauffeur agreed to let me walk around, but drove next to me at 2 mph, with a gun!

From then on, I was invited to all family weddings and holidays. But, due to the distance, I never grew close to anyone except the Philadelphia relatives, Inge, Steven, and Peter. I was, however, very close to The List members.

When I was in Cambodia, I woke up to read the news that Susan's son had committed suicide. While everyone else was eating breakfast, I stayed in my room and cried. That's how close I felt to Susan, even though we had only met in person once.

For my husband Peter's 50th birthday, he wanted to go to Israel which was perfect timing for me. There I met three members of The List: Judy Montel, Ruth (both of whom I had met previously in Boston), and Nathalie who I had never met before. I enjoyed meeting all of them. The highlight was going into Ruth's bomb shelter where she had painted rockets being fired at Lebanon.

This was a truly life changing experience, and I found Israel to be fascinating. It strengthened my ties with Judaism. As my uncle Gerhardt was supposedly dying, I put a prayer for him in the Western Wall, and he survived.

I spent about 10 years being obsessed with the Holocaust. I made a family tree on my father's side going back seven generations. I also discovered the details of who they were, what had happened to them, and exactly how some were murdered.

I decided to visit my father on his birthday. His birthday present was the family tree, and a binder full of our family's documents. It was probably the worst birthday present he ever got. He started by looking at the family tree. His response was that his mother's name was not Dreyfus (which it was) and that he was going to take a nap. He never took a close look at the tree, and totally ignored the binder.

I was leaving the next day. My dilemma was whether to leave the tree & binder behind or take it with me. I immediately put the question out to The List. They helped me to decide to leave it behind. I'll never know if he looked at it but I think he was too curious to not have looked at it. After his death, when I cleaned out his house, the things I had left were gone, as was any evidence of his Jewish identity.

I went back to Boston and started a Holocaust book club which continued for many years. We are all still friends. Although anyone could join, it was the 2g's (Second Generation) and survivors who stayed in the group. I began to feel like I was an expert in Holocaust studies and literature. I was also a tour guide for 10–15 years at the New England Holocaust Memorial. I didn't need training. I knew everything, and there wasn't a single question I could not answer. Every book I read, every movie I saw was about the Holocaust. I seemed to be under a spell until...

I went with the Terezin Music Association to Prague. Although we were there to attend the music festival and see Prague, we were also there to visit the Terezin concentration camp. I knew so much about that camp in particular, that I knew it would be one of the easiest ones to visit. I would never have considered going to Auschwitz.

I was wrong. Terezin was not as easy to visit as I had thought. We toured the camp, seeing everything I had already known about, but I was not prepared for the crematorium. The Terezin Music Association came with Boston Symphony violinists. As we entered the crematorium, I was handed a piece of paper which I recognized as being the Kaddish. There were unlit candles sitting at the entrance of the oven, and the violins were playing. We were each supposed to light one candle and I couldn't handle it. I ran from the room and had a total meltdown. After a while, I gathered my strength to go back and light my candle. That's what broke the spell. I was freed from my Holocaust obsession. No more books, movies, etc. I was done.

I shared this experience with The List, and they shared their experiences of visiting concentration camps. All of them had emotional experiences as well.

A few years later, I was offered the opportunity to go on a free trip sponsored by the City of Frankfurt. I was curious to see the places that were relevant to my family. I saw our family factory that was stolen by the Nazis, probably worth a billion dollars now. I couldn't even get in. I saw a dozen apartment buildings that my family had owned. Some were luxurious, others were rebuilt poorly after having been bombed. In the Jewish Museum

I found the front door of our family home in medieval times. Outside, there was a long wall with small plaques, bearing the names of people from Frankfurt who had been murdered. There I saw the names of the murdered Rothschilds, a family that had intermarried with our own.

I went to a service at our family synagogue, miraculously undamaged due to the proximity of their (stolen Jewish) homes to the synagogue. Throughout the trip, I stayed in touch with The List whose members gave me feedback.

I was asked to speak at a German school, and they sent me to my father's school. I told the story of my family in a room that my father had probably sat in fifty years earlier. The school still maintained records of all their students, so I saw my father's records. Two things stood out. My father's birthday matched his birth certificate. Then I knew that our family celebrations of my father's birthday had always been on the wrong day. Another interesting fact was that he dropped out of the school in 1934, the same year my grandfather was arrested by the Gestapo, yet Jews still had not been denied education that year.

While on this trip, there was too much information for me to process. Upon my return, I went to the New England Holocaust Memorial and waited for my tour to arrive. I began crying and realized how much antisemitism had affected my life.

In 2019, it became apparent that antisemitism was rising at an alarming speed throughout the world. Jews were being killed again, and the whole world seemed to want the destruction of Israel. I decided to do something about it. I started a Facebook group called "Action Against Anti-Semitism". Currently it has about 1,100 members. We do exactly what the name says, fight antisemitism wherever we see it. I want to help ensure that the same thing that happened to my family will never happen again.

My husband Pete accompanied me on all my travels and was always there for support. He accepted my obsession with the Holocaust. After seven years of suffering from a variety of illnesses, he died in 2016 at the age of 59. I was his caretaker with much difficulty. I had cancer and other illnesses and injuries as well. Throughout this period The List was very supportive. Just last week I was informed by a cardiologist that I have a hole in my heart. That's the hole that Pete left.

My Cyber Family

Although it was an email group of approximately 60 people, I met about 15 of them in person. I always thought of Hanna as the mother of our group.

Not because she was older, but she seemed to be the glue who helped keep us together. I was fortunate to have met her and found that she was every bit as wonderful as I thought.

I met Laurie on three occasions and felt particularly close to her. Once, on the first night of Passover, my husband had a heart attack in Philadelphia. Laurie, who lived in D.C., offered to come. I knew the Passover traffic would be unbearable and I declined her offer. Denise invited me to meet her when she was on Cape Cod. I drove there feeling a little uncomfortable to be staying with a family I had never met. The whole family was wonderful. Denise and I had so much to say to each other. Our conversation was an extension of The List conversation.

I met many others. I also became close with many I never met, and still hope to meet. There are too many to name. We are moving into the next phase. Two List members have died, and we all know that our turn is coming. I know that The List is strong enough and our bonds are so close, that we will be supporting each other until the end of our lives.

Paul Foldes
The List Creator's Story

Introduction

Descending upon the New York runway with its wheels stuck, the plane made an emergency landing, stopping somewhere on the tarmac. There were fire trucks on the runway. I had spent most of the flight trying to be a "good boy", melting into my seat, and doing what I was told. After all, during our escape from Communist Hungary I had learned that life, literally, often depended on doing just that. It wasn't the most uplifting memory of my first sight of the United States, nor the best introduction to freedom for a ten-and-a-half-year-old Hungarian refugee boy, whose family had fled during the Hungarian revolution. But freedom it was, as I would learn during the next few months.

There was a lot that we managed to leave behind. Communism. The terror of being informed upon by our neighbors. The grey existence of life in a country whose economy was being mishandled and destroyed by the Stalinist regime. As I began to get used to the American freedom, I tried to put as many of those bad memories as I could behind me and concentrate upon my new life. But there was one thing that I couldn't leave behind. The fact that I was the son of two Holocaust survivors. My Second Generation (2g) identity was imbedded in me and would continue to be a major part of me no matter where I was, and what I did. For years, I was busy with everyday life, school, professional training, making a living, being a husband, father, and son. But eventually, that part of my life caught up with me, and I realized how much I could use the support of my peers, other 2gs. It was then that I decided to create The List. But that is far in the future. To get there, one must first begin with the past.

Family History Before My Birth

I have relatively little knowledge of my family's history prior to my birth, as I grew up as an only child, with parents who didn't volunteer much. Whenever they made any reference to their pre-Holocaust life in my presence, the degree of sadness and emotions that permeated their words made me extremely reluctant to ask them any questions, for fear of causing them more pain. As my father was dying from cancer, I tried to get him to talk about his life, but he waived me off with the words: "take care of your mother". Unfortunately, I grew up alone, with no grandparents, other than my mother's father who died when I was eight, an uncle I did not meet until I was 22 and visited in Israel, and no aunts or first cousins who could fill me in on family history. Similarly, I was also reluctant to ask my uncle and one second cousin I knew as a young adult, for fear of bringing back painful memories. I also feared what would happen to my own emotional state if they would actually talk to me about these things.

What information I have I got indirectly, either through casual reference in conversation or overhearing things mentioned while talking with the few surviving relatives left. And as I was so fearful of broaching the subject that I don't have much understanding of what really went on, only the most skeletal details of events. The extent of my fear of hurting family members by asking, and my own fear of being hurt while learning what happened to them and their families, is manifested by my not having had the courage to visit the exhibits on the upper floors of the US Holocaust Museum in Washington DC where I have visited numerous times. I have only been to the first-floor auditorium for events accompanying my mother, who lived near me in the suburbs of Washington DC.

The only thing I know about my parent's lives before the Holocaust was that they apparently had happy childhoods, with many activities and friends. They were also very good and vigorous dancers, something I learned while watching them do the Czardas and Waltzes at gatherings and occasions.

My mother was the beautiful, only child of a prosperous, loving, doting father. Together with two other men, he was a partner in a chain of three haberdasher stores in Miskolc and Debrecen and survived the Holocaust by being conscripted to a forced labor camp in Ukraine. When he restarted his store after returning from Ukraine, the Communists in Hungary confiscated it.

His daughter, my mother, was an Olympic gymnast finalist, chosen to represent Hungary in the 1936 Olympics, but was not allowed to compete because she was Jewish. She and her mother were deported to Auschwitz where my grandmother was murdered. Having always been very close to her mother, my mother missed her terribly after the war. The only thing I know about my mother's wartime experiences in Auschwitz was that she lost a piece of her finger in an accident, while working for Krupp in an underground munitions manufacturing facility, and that she survived the death march from Auschwitz to Mauthausen.

My father's father, one of six brothers, was a farmer near Hejobaba, which probably motivated my father to get a PhD in Animal Husbandry.

That was no small accomplishment in 1937 when fewer PhD's were around in any discipline. It was an even bigger accomplishment in Hungary, where from 1934 onward, universities began applying quotas to Jews, severely limiting their opportunities to enroll and attend. His younger brother by just a few years was banned from attending university.

I have a picture of him in a cavalry officers' uniform, sword and all. I know that he loved riding horses, and had mentioned riding bareback on the farm, early in the morning. Whenever we drove by a fenced field with horses in the country, he invariably stopped, went over to the fence, and if lucky, enticed a horse to come over to be petted on the nose. That was the only time I saw him light up, except for the times he would dance with my mother.

I know little of his family beyond these facts. I do know that before the war, his father and some of his brothers were quite entrepreneurial, one owning a tractor manufacturing factory which went bankrupt during the Depression. My father found one of their tractors on display in the Budapest mechanical truck/tractor museum. Before his premature death at age 77, he proudly showed it off to his too-young-to-appreciate grandson on their last family trip to Hungary together in 1991.

Growing up I had the fortune of knowing one of my father's uncles, who also survived forced labor in Ukraine. He was my favorite person. I admired his out-of-the-box thinking, feisty non-group think nature, and inherited much of it. He was trained as an engineer in Berlin, was warm, witty, resilient, smart, and successfully outfoxed the Communists who confiscated his farm. He raised pigs in his backyard to help make ends meet as the local communist party officials were severely trying to harm his well-being. He survived loss of his first wife and daughter in the Holocaust, and the death of his wonderful second wife after a relatively long marriage, all while maintaining a spunk that I inherited from him. At age 88 he came to visit his nephews in the United States and Israel, picked up design ideas for an egg collecting machine, which he then sold to the local communist collective manager. He never gave up!

My Story

Both of my parents had been married before and lost their first spouses in the war. It appears that my mother married in 1943, and her first husband, who was in a Wallenberg safe house, was caught when he went out to get food, and was never seen again. About my father's family I know even less. He never spoke about his first wife, his son, or his parents, all of whom perished in the Holocaust.

My parents married in 1946, after returning home to Miskolc to find that none of their families had survived. They had known each other well before the German invasion, and in fact, my father had even been a contender for my mother's hand in marriage before she chose to marry her first husband. My mother was very disciplined. She was the "strong one" in the family, constantly having to support my father's flailing confidence and calm his emotional upsets.

Like many survivors, my parents soon started a family. I was born in April 1947 and named after my mother's first husband who perished in the Holocaust. As the first child born to a woman in that town who survived the death camps, I was considered a "miracle" child. Why? Given the extreme emaciation they endured, no one knew how soon, if ever, would these women be able to bear children.

I don't really remember much about my Hungarian childhood. Maybe I've blocked it out as it was such a difficult period in everyone's lives. Living in Hungary under Communism was unlike what anyone growing up in the Free World can imagine. The best description is what I have read by Anne Applebaum, the Washington Post's foreign correspondent in her book *Iron Curtain: The Crushing of Eastern Europe, 1944–1956*. I remember a lot of fear as we were living under Stalin, and my childhood coincided with Stalin's reign of terror. My mother and father lived in constant fear of neighbors informing on them, and their being sent to a Gulag. What would happen to me then? For example, when the father of one of my friends disappeared, I was told that he was away on a trip overseas. I do remember nearly being killed during the revolution by a Russian soldier doing a house-to-house search. In short, whatever I went through in the United States afterwards, it was paradise compared to my early childhood in Hungary.

I escaped from Hungary with my parents, crossing the Iron Curtain on foot on the night of December 12, 1956. I was nine-and-a-half years old, the oldest of six children (the youngest was six months old) and six adults in our group, being led by gypsy smugglers who lived near the border. At one point before that, I remember cowering in a corner of a cabin on a train as we were trying to escape, while a Russian soldier decided whether to arrest us. We were lucky. He didn't, and thus we were not among the 600 people that they eventually took off that train. At another point during our escape, we spent a few hours in a haystack at 2:00 am on a moonlit night while flicking pebbles at a guard tower, checking whether it was manned, before trying to pass. Eventually, we rode in a truck to Vienna, and were dropped off at the Rothschild Hospital, where a hall was set up to process the stream of refugees arriving after the violent crushing of the Hungarian Revolution by the Russian army.

After a month, the authorities found room for us in a former US Army camp near Salzburg that was empty after Austria became neutralized in 1955 and occupation troops left. We spent 10 months there awaiting our fate, seeking entry into any country that would give us a place to live. My mother pushed for going to the United States, if given the chance, as she was liberated by the US Army. My father preferred Israel as his brother emigrated there in 1949, just before the Iron Curtain descended, making emigration impossible.

In the refugee camp near Salzburg, we were segregated into a separate building. As Jews, our fellow Hungarian antisemitic refugee camp mates wanted to kill us. Antisemitism has never been far from my life experience.

After 10 months of statelessness, we were fortunate to have been admitted in the United States as political refugees. But admission did not yet mean security. During our first two years in America there was no assurance that we could stay, until the FBI checked our bona fides and we were granted a "green card". Only three years after receiving that "green card" could we become naturalized American citizens, which we proudly became at first opportunity afforded on the calendar.

We arrived in New York City on October 28, 1957 on a chartered DC3 plane. The trip had taken 63 hours, because due to mechanical problems, it made three emergency landings on the way. On our first night in United States, we were greeted by our hosts in the USA – the only people my parents knew from Hungary – who had been kind enough to take on the responsibility of sponsoring us, guaranteeing that we would not become wards of the State. As they drove us around Times Square that first night, overcome by the sight of the tall buildings and bright lights, I threw up in the car. The Budapest I grew up in had been dark and grey, due to the energy shortages and devastating economic conditions under Communism. All these lights were something very new, and somewhat overwhelming.

In November 1957, less than two weeks of our arrival, I was enrolled in the 5th grade at PS158 in Manhattan, (based on my chronological age) notwithstanding the fact that I had not attended 3rd or 4th grades due to time spent in transit. As I did not speak any English, I basically skipped 5th grade as well, during which time I memorized twenty words a day from a dictionary. I didn't start putting words together and learn to speak English until the summer of 1958 when I attended a Jewish charity-run camp, where I had to speak English to be able to co-exist with fellow campers.

My parents didn't have the luxury of waiting months before communicating in English. Within two or three months of our arrival, both found jobs that would require them to speak some English, my father as an elevator operator (manual elevators in those days) and my mother as a payroll clerk. It was the fourth time my father had started life anew after losing his entire family, having his back broken in Dachau, being stripped of his property, first by the Nazis and then by the Communists, and having to take on new working-class identity as a meat inspector, as someone with a doctorate in Animal Husbandry was considered a threat to the Stalinist regime.

Seeing his intelligence, my father was soon moved to an office where he became an accounting clerk. As children of well-established parents, my parents' childhood had been that of privilege. Mine, however, was that of a child of two office clerks with menial pay, frequent layoffs, and numerous slights at work by colleagues who looked down on them. Their economic and work insecurities, stemming from being laid off frequently, coupled with feelings of inferiority due to lack of language and cultural familiarity, understandably resulted in frustrations that permeated our household. Such insecurities, and their negative consequences, have also been present for most of my life.

My regular schooling restarted in 1958 when I entered 6th grade (5th was a space holder as I didn't understand a word said by teacher or other kids). That was followed by middle school where I gained a small gang of friends who introduced me to American sports like baseball and football, all new to me as I grew up playing soccer.

In 1960 I became Bar Mitzvah to the great joy of my parents. With little money or knowledge of customs, they put on a small reception in our tiny one-bedroom apartment in Astoria, inviting my Public School teachers, as was the custom in Hungary – some of whom came!

I received two memorable gifts, a bicycle and my mother's Doxa watch that she wore during our journey from Hungary to America. In 1962, I was admitted to Stuyvesant High School, one of New York City's highly competitive math and science high schools. I thrived there, thanks to the help of very understanding and supportive teachers, who, despite my having skipped three grades, allowed me to finagle my way into advanced placement classes, and provided me with a first-class education. If it wasn't for two of them, I would not have known how to apply both to college, and for scholarships.

From Stuyvesant High School I proceeded to New York University (NYU) from which I graduated with an Electrical Engineering degree. I had no "classic college experience" of dorm life, or rah-rah sports games, as

I was a commuter, working two jobs and helping my parents with household chores during college. I had chosen to major in Engineering to qualify for scholarships that were more available in that field during post Sputnik era. In truth, however, I had little innate interest in the subject.

While interning at IBM during the summer between my junior and senior years at NYU, I learned that IBM and some other major corporations had Patent Attorney Trainee Programs in which science and engineering graduates with aptitude for law, were given daytime jobs while having their law school tuition paid to study law at night. I jumped at the chance to get one of those relatively few slots, and applied for, but wasn't accepted to, the IBM program. Nevertheless, I received offers from several corporations for their Patent Attorney Trainee programs.

I ended up going to Georgetown Law Center at night, while working for General Motors patent section during the day as a Patent Attorney Trainee with my tuition paid, along with an engineer's salary. Unfortunately, I was laid off in my first year during the recession of 1970. Luckily, I had applied for and was accepted for a Patent Examiner position in the US Patent Office before graduating from NYU and had a position which also involved working during the day while attending law school at night. Tuition was paid for relevant courses if one agreed to work for the Government for five years.

At the Patent Office I was unluckily assigned to a very boring, time intensive unit, where I spent two painfully frustrating years while earning a good salary. Fortunately, during this time, I met my future wife at Georgetown Law, who then steered me to a life-transforming opportunity to be a Legal Assistant at the Federal Trade Commission where she was working at that time. She facilitated both of us getting these coveted slots, and we both had very substantial and rewarding assignments there as Legal Assistants, even before we graduated and passed the Bar. She was the assistant to the General Counsel, and I was an assistant on several landmark cases that gave me great satisfaction. My time at the Federal Trade Commission began a lifelong interest in public service which continues until today.

After graduating, we married and started our family. This brought a great deal of happiness to my parents who saw this culmination of all their sacrifices. Finally, new life and family were being re-established after the great losses they suffered during the Holocaust.

Life, however, is not static. My life changed radically in 1983 when my marriage ended abruptly, and I became a single father of a five-year-old son. At the same time, I was financially stressed. I had left the Federal Trade Commission a few years earlier and entered the business world just as the greatest recession since the Great Depression was beginning. It took me a while, but I managed to rebuild my life. My "survivor" gene and firsthand experience as a refugee-immigrant, helped me start anew.

Just when I thought that things were going more smoothly, a series of calamities set me back again. My savings were embezzled by a Ponzi schemer in 1990, and my father died of esophageal cancer at age 77 in 1991, like so many survivors who died prematurely of cancer, as I later learned. On top of that, the Great Recession continued to severally stress my professional/business life. I prevailed, striving to be best single father I could be to my son, while also taking on the role of my mother's prime emotional support and caregiver.

I persevered through the 1990s, but recall very little, other than pain and numbness. During that time, I also met my partner of last 25 years through close friends who lied to each of us. She had been told by her best friend that I was financially stable, while I was told by her best friend's father, my professional mentor/and pending business partner, that she wanted to move back to the east coast from San Francisco, where she was living at the time. In truth, she absolutely had no intention of moving, and I was financially unstable. My father just died, and I was doing the best I could as a single parent, with no support or understanding from my parents. Neither of them believed in divorce, even if it had not happened at my instigation, and were indirectly criticizing my parenting, which was also not in my control. We met on a blind date at a concert hall, where I promptly fell asleep during the first half of the concert (it was modern music). We then had dinner and talked for a few hours after the concert, after which, as they say, "the rest is history".

My partner, who in a former life was a K-5 teacher, but didn't have children of her own, found a groove with my son who was then 13. Together, they provided the stability in my life that I sorely lacked since my divorce.

She helped me raise a very loving, caring son, who later became a terrific father with many of the attributes I didn't possess, including being more laid back than I ever was. Not surprising, given that the rap on me has always been: "He takes everything so seriously, why doesn't he ease up and get a life?". Fortunately, my son survived my seriousness in parenting him. I was always the over-concerned parent, just as my parents had been towards me during my childhood. That was quite understandable, given what they went through, first under the Nazis, and then, under Stalin's reign of terror. Add to that the challenges of being stateless, and then having to cope in a new country without speaking the language, or knowing the culture, and you rarely have a recipe for easygoing parents.

I used to joke that I was going to have a "first childhood" while raising my son, but that didn't turn out as hoped. Rather, that has been happening as I have the privilege of being closely involved with the development of the children that he and his wife have provided me with, my wonderful grandson and granddaughter. Only now have I finally begun to experience what a normal childhood looks and feels like, finally healing the breach in my family that had been caused by the Holocaust.

Starting after my divorce in the early1980s and continuing for the next two decades, I was a solo, independent, commercial real estate broker, something that allowed me to care for my mother as she aged, and be there for my son as well, all while making a living. As a primary caregiver to both generations, I was able to fulfill my responsibilities without work interfering in those tasks. Luckily, I continued to do so until my mother passed away at home when she was 82, following a series of strokes, and my son successfully graduated from college in 2000. It was during these years, while focusing on caring for the generation before me and that after me, that I also began giving some thought to my generation, and particularly those who belonged to the "Second Generation" like me. That was one of the factors that brought me to create "The List".

Genesis of the List

Before there was "The List" there was "the idea". And before there was "the idea", there was the recognition of "the need". How did I realize there was "a need"? And what brought me to go about meeting "that need" in the way I did? Here is the story.

Actually, several factors merged together in order to help me create "The List". The first began during the late 1980s, before the Internet existed as we know it today. At that time, a series of private online forums (BBS's) and communities run by individuals began to take shape. Each of them was centered around a particular interest and was connected through an informal network. The second occurred in 1990, when a friend took me to a 12-step meeting where I first had a chance to experience the power of a "peer to peer" self-help group. As I had slowly become aware of my uniqueness as a member of the "Second Generation", I immediately began looking for a similar "peer to peer" type Second Generation group in the Washington Area where I lived. After attending meetings of several, the local ones I found did not satisfy my personal needs. So, I began thinking about broadening my search beyond my immediate surroundings. I turned to the online world where I came across a number of peer-to-peer self-support groups on different platforms, first on CompuServe then on the emerging AOL.

Together, those realizations and experiences led me to establish the Second Generation List, aka "The List". I initially established it on a network of private online Computer Bulletin Board System (BBS) forums, a means of group communication predating the public internet system. When the Internet as we know it started to emerge in the early 90s, first as a network of email and text-only based channels, and later as a graphical interface based "web", I began migrating The List to the "open", just gestating Internet.

Information about the existence of The List became known through "word of mouse" when it migrated to Shamash, a Jewish Internet platform that carried The List as a free service. Shamash's directory of channels made it possible for members of the Second Generation worldwide to find The List and join the online community where they could establish connections beyond their physically immediate network of family and friends. As word of its existence spread, The List grew organically, and relatively quickly.

The Second Generation's need for mutual support became self-evident as people joined The List from North and South America, Europe, and Israel. Many of the members quickly developed emotional ties with each other. I was no exception. The ability to share the stories of our lives provided great sustenance to me, as I hadn't realized how much our experiences as children of Survivors had affected us. Books by Helen Epstein and other Second Generation researchers were already reporting about finding some general similarities among members of that group, and the dynamics on The List further strengthened these conclusions. The conclusions we reached during various discussions, and the emotional experiences that we underwent during our cathartic interchanges, provided me and others on The List, with a great deal of comfort, particularly when coming across kindred souls.

However, it wasn't all good. As the internet became more familiar and began experiencing inter-community turmoil, The List, too, exhibited quite uncomfortable "flaming". The viciousness of the messages being posted by a few of the members caused me, and some of the others, great pain and anguish. There was so much "yelling" in writing that it became exhausting to read, not only for me, but for other members as well. Consequently, we agreed to put the previously unmoderated List on "moderated" status, with me acting as moderator, which was no easy task. Basically, it meant that I had to read each and every message intended for posting before allowing it to be posted, to make sure that it was not purposefully inflammatory. At some point, this cost me up to 45 minutes a day of painful emotional experiences. So painful, that it is already hard for me to remember the nitty-gritty of many of the arguments and noisy discussions, and I am just left with the general hollow feeling of having had to deal with everyone's anger (against a situation, against each other, not against me as moderator) all the time.

Finally, in 1999, it became too overwhelming for me. Like many in such situations, I felt that I was experiencing burnout, and to rest my soul, I first relinquished my role as moderator, and ultimately left The List to have some peace and quiet in my life. Second Generation communication is good, but there is a thing as too much noise while communicating, making the whole experience more painful than uplifting. In retrospect, that is probably what happened to me.

For twenty years I didn't look to see what happened to my creation. Had I done so, I would have learned that The List continued and evolved into an online "family" with its ups and downs. But it had indeed become a family, supportive of its members as they passed along their life journeys. Boy, could I have used such sustenance during my 20-year absence!

When this book was being contemplated, a List member who had orchestrated the group's latest move to a different Internet platform, got in touch with me to ask whether I wished to contribute to this book. Hearing about The List's continued existence and family-like evolution over the years, I promptly asked to rejoin and was most warmly welcomed back to the fold. The List was now back in my life.

Epilogue

The list has been a great satisfaction to me. It allowed many members of the Second Generation from so many places on the globe to easily come together online for the first time. It provided a safe (admission by request only), private place where they could sort out their feelings and support each other among empathetic peers who had undergone similar, and at times, stressful experiences during their childhoods.

Like another peer-to-peer 12 step network to which I belong, that has existed in various forms for three quarters of a century, The List has given me the support to deal with and recover from the trauma that my parents transmitted to me, through no fault of their own. More than anything else, The List provided me with the opportunity to be of service to others, something I continue to get great satisfaction from doing to this day!

Martin Herskovitz
How the List Transformed My Life

Introduction – Finding Roots

My house was too fierce a place to ever serve as a home. First, there were too many walls. Barriers were everywhere, communication was impossible. Second, despite all these walls, our house never really provided shelter, as if the home had no emotional roof. I felt exposed, vulnerable, and unsafe. I don't blame my parents for trying to build a home and failing. My mother was a Holocaust survivor. My father was left to live with his grandparents when his parents and three other siblings (one older sister, two younger) immigrated to America. These traumas which were foisted on them, prevented them from creating a true home for us. They were able to build only a shell of a home that left us without a true anchor to build our lives.

> Rootlessness
> My father, aged 12
> Arrived in America
> 6 years after his family,
> left him behind.
> Upon his arrival he refused to kiss the unfamiliar woman
> who met him at the pier.
> It was his mother.
> I imagine that until he got readjusted to his new family
> that he felt between homes, rootless.
> His eyes would lose their focus every once in a while
> (like they did as a five-year old
> trying to remember what his mother looked like)
> until he forced himself to grow up quickly
> and not need a mother at all.
> I think about my father's legacy
> wandering alone
> trying to decide
> how much of a home
> I can learn not to need
> And how much of a home
> I will be able to build

For me, being a Second Generation has been a modern-day Mark of Cain. I have been unable, as I have imagined my father also being unable, to find a true feeling of belonging, of finding my place. My life is a constant search for looking to belong, and at the same time, running away from belonging, terrified of being abandoned.

But there are times, moments of grace, when I have felt I belonged. Places I have felt safe enough to express my feelings, express my fears. The Second Generation listserv that I joined in the end of 1999 was such a place. I found a virtual home for a few short years until I moved on, or perhaps The List moved on. But those few years influenced me then and influence me now, as I try to build my life anew. This is my story and its story, and how we intertwined and then grew apart.

My Life Before I was Born – The Holocaust

A child of Holocaust survivors seldom has a life of their own. We are often named for someone, or more than one person, and we are brought into the world to replace those souls who were lost, dozens of souls.

> Berries
> I remember the ceremony, as a child,
> in the lengthening shade of the mulberry tree,
> as the Kibbutz elders read the names.
> Their names,
> names that had become ours.
> Names like a breeze
> that wafted upwards through the tendriled
> green mulberries.
> Names like the shadow that grew long
> with day's end.
> Late that summer I would return to the tree
> to pick these mulberries from the ground
> their sweetness embittered with dust,
> unaware of the names that had lodged in my soul
> like the tiny hard seeds of a mulberry.

The path of my life was determined before I was born. I was intended to replace those dozens of souls who were never spoken about, never grieved. If I could have done a good enough job to replace them, then my parents wouldn't have to ever think about those others, would be able to pretend that they needn't be mourned.

How The List Transformed My Life

In order to understand me fully, we should start in 1898 when Nettie Jakubowitz left the United States to return to Seredne and marry Abraham Herskovitz, but this is an essay and not a saga. So, I will not begin then, but will tell my story, beginning in the year 1944, the year my mother and my father turned 21, half a world apart, my mother in Seredne, my father in a Navy Training base in San Diego.

In the beginning of 1944, my father had enlisted in the Navy against his father's wishes and had finished training as a radio operator. He was on his way to Leyte Gulf to take part in the largest Naval battle ever fought.

My mother was still in Seredne where life had taken a turn for the worse with the overthrow of the Horthy Government by Hitler. In spring 1944, the Nazi army, returning from defeat in Russia, occupied Hungary and installed a puppet government that acceded to the German request to begin exterminating Hungarian Jewry. The Hungarians began transporting Jews to "ghettos" – which were little more than shantytowns near the railway stations – in preparation for transport to Auschwitz-Birkenau.

The deportations from Seredne occurred on the day of the Seder. The holiday which commemorates the salvation of the Jews became the day when their destruction began. Even more ironically, the day which was meant to represent the day when firstborns were endangered, became the day when the firstborns actually survived, and the younger siblings were sent to their death, being too young to serve as laborers.

Seder Night, 1944 Birkenau
The firstborn of Velvel and Feige Gruen was spared on Passover Eve 5704,
But all her brothers and sisters were killed.
The firstborn of Lipa and Masha Tarnowicz was spared on Passover Eve 5704,
But thousands of others exterminated.
Why the terrible deliverance of that night?
Why did the Angel of Death just stay, just stay
Was it that their prayers were whispered and not cried aloud.
Or that there was no hyssop in Auschwitz 1944,
And no blood,
Just ashes and smoke.

On that Passover Day, all the Jews of Seredne were lined up and counted. The Jews were asked to stand at attention, in formation, while the lists were consulted, and the numbers confirmed. They all stood stock still except for one.

Pixieman

They called him Pixieman
Because his forehead sloped up in a funny way
And he laughed a lot,
And he had long thick shoelaces, so he could tie them
And the bows would flop on the ground.
When he did errands for his mother
they would run after him yelling "Pixieman, Pixieman",
But he would just smile
When the Nazis marched them from the ghetto to the train station,
Pixieman got startled by the gnarling dogs or perhaps shouts of the soldiers
and bolted into the forest.
A dozen soldiers were sent
while the rest of the town had to wait on the road facing forward
out of the corner of her eye my aunt saw him being dragged,
sobbing and shivering back into the line.
They continued on, Pixieman shuffling forward,
Eyes lowered, his shoelaces caked in mud,
Trembling.
His trembling stopped, with death,
a few days later, at Birkenau

The 3,000 some Jews of Seredne were taken to the Brickyard in Ungvar (Uzhgorod today). There wasn't enough food and water, and disease was rampant. The residents of Ungvar hastened the Nazis to transport the Jews away as quickly as possible, and by Shavuot (Pentecost), the Ghetto was already gone, all the Jews deported. My mother and her family arrived in Auschwitz a day or two before the Holiday. Every narrative of the arrival to Birkenau has a description of the selection process and each description has its own trauma. There are stories of whispered warning, last minute providences, of chance salvations. Our family has that too. My Aunt Esther was helping her sister carry a child in the line. One of the women guards, a Czech woman, whispered to her to put the child down, to give her back to the mother. She did and her life was saved. But my mother's sister was told by my mother and her sister just the opposite – to help their mother with the children. Whispered advice, last minute improvidence and a life lost. It is the one story that weighed upon my mother. The one story she told.

History

My mother has no history,
Only labyrinths of possibilities,

radiating from junctures in time.
"What if, on the causeway,
we had pulled Hensche with us,
and piled her a mound of gravel on which to stand,
propping her between our shoulders,
pinching her when the officer neared
to stand erect.
She might have lived."
But instead my Mother and her sister sent her to the other side
to the children huddled about their Mother.
"We didn't know, we couldn't know."
But even so,
Would fate have dragged Hensche from the furnace
Or would she have plunged all three to oblivion.
For in a place where death is imminent,
And survival a chance occurrence
There is no surety, there is no surety,
And destiny tempted turns easily vengeful.
The paths not taken are not overgrown with green
But alleyways of blackest cinder
burrows of swirling dusts,
Barbed and spiny.
And when memory allows
My mother travels these passages
And bows her head against imagined blows.

My mother spent an eternity in Auschwitz in the C Lager, waiting for her fate to be decided, A few days, or maybe weeks later, she was sent to spend another eternity in KZ Walldorf near Frankfurt, filling the holes and ruts in the Frankfurt airport runaways, Then, when the U.S. Army drew too close, she was sent to spend another lifetime eternity in Ravensbrück, which had deteriorated into barely controlled chaos, ravaged by typhoid, littered with the dead and dying. At Ravensbrück she was ransomed by the Swedish Red Cross in the spring of 1945. Of the various lifetimes my mother has spoken little. She didn't think that her story was especially significant.

<u>Silence</u>
My mother has never spoken of what happened during the War,
and never will.
Her aunt gave a video testimony

> What she has to say, she said,
> has been told
> over and over,
> just the number on the arm differs.
> It is only now, when she can no longer speak,
> That I realize that the silence has wounded
> more than words

We have established the setting into which I was born. A world of two souls ravaged by traumas, seeking refuge, seeking a home. That home that they would try to build want to build with us, the children to come. The children who will become the focus of their lives, but ironically, they will be unable to love.

Rising From the Ashes

My father's family was the closest family my mother had in the world, so after a year of rehabilitation in the Swedish countryside, my mother went to Chicago to stay with them. She was treated horrendously by her aunt and uncle. First, she was terribly resented for having survived, while their beloved parents, of saintly memory, were slaughtered: "Why did you survive and not they?" She was made to serve as a domestic in the house, to cook, clean and watch over the children who were just a few years younger than she. They made fun of her that she didn't know English, couldn't read and write. No one was particularly interested in hearing about her ordeal. Her cousins would say things like, "We suffered too. Did you know that we couldn't get sugar or kosher meat?" So, my mother stopped talking about the horrors. The only one of the children who treated her nicely was my father. Perhaps because he too had been an immigrant once, he suffered the embarrassment of not knowing the language, of being the outsider in a new and strange world.

My father recognized a kindred soul, another of the walking wounded, posttraumatic, afraid of intimacy and renewing bonds, but even needier of a relationship to fill the emptiness. They were a couple who desperately needed each connection, the feeling of family. And yet, they were too wounded to truly communicate and relate. They were not loving enough to create a loving family. In some way, it was a perfect match. In other ways, it was a relationship doomed to failure, as both were unable to provide the intimacy and emotional security that the other craved and needed in order to heal.

How The List Transformed My Life   99

My mother and father got married in December 1946, about half a year after my mother first set foot on Ellis Island. They immediately began building the family that they thought would heal their wounds. They gave little thought to the fact that they, still in the throes of tragedy, still trying to piece their shattered psyches together again, were not quite ready to build a family.

Renewal
Jerusalem after the snow,
almond trees blanketed in frost.
I watched their branches swirl in the gusts,
showering petals that could not hold fast.
It is cruel to bloom in the winter,
When one's sap is turgid and sour,
translucent petals exposed to the shivering sleet.
What fruits will be brought forth from these,
thick husked and bitter no doubt.
And when stillness comes, of what do these blossoms dream?
Of warm summer breezes and shimmering red flowers,
and hummingbirds craning their sparkling neck
to sip of their fragrant nectar, perhaps.
But theirs is to bloom while the hummingbirds sleep,
impelled by some impassive force of nature, bent on renewal,
to put forth these tiny pale flowers,
in the midst of the maelstrom

In 1948, my sister Nancy was born, three years later Brenda arrived, and I was born in 1955. Our purpose in life was to fill the void, the aftermath of the traumas. It was an impossible task, and we failed miserably

Pharaoh's Cow
I am part of a war unfinished
a war that will never be finished,
its dead unburied, unmourned.
I am part of lives concealed,
a syllable in a secret unwhispered,
sealed in a chamber of pain.
I am part of a chasm of need,
its famine unsated,
Like the cow in Pharaoh's dream,
devouring fatted heifers,
gaunt with dissatisfaction.

Each of the siblings took on a persona in order to deal with their failure to cure our parents, to take away their trauma, to become good enough for their love, or if not love, at least their attention.

My oldest sister, Nancy, born a year and a couple of months after my parent's marriage, became the hero child. She tried to be the "perfect" child. She felt a strong responsibility for our parents, who were unable to love us and take care of us due to their trauma, and she took on the role as parent to her younger siblings.

In the shadow of the placating perfect child, my other sister and I became "lost children", running away from expectations. We learned that the best way to survive is to be invisible and "blend into the woodwork"; to have little expectations of family or of ourselves.

Shattered Dreams
Dreams were the enemy
Because they looked for ends and beginnings
In a world where middleness survived.
In a world where time needed to meld into
Daysmonthsyears
Dreams lengthened the minutes
And drew the notch ever tighter
And all the dreams they hadn't allowed
Were bequeathed to us.
And I became a child of expectation
Presaged and impendent
Who ran from the dreams surrounding.
But dreams return, on wings of hope,
to shatter ever stronger.

Yet the expectation was always there, and we failed to find the love and acceptance because my parents were unable to provide it. In our family, I took the role of the Lost Child. The Lost Child comes into a dysfunctional family after a few children have been born and understands or feels the strain the family is under. As a result, they try to minimize their demands on their parents and siblings. I tried to make myself as unseen as possible, so not to add to the strain my family was under. As a result, I was overlooked. But this leaves these children feeling lonely, rejected, and isolated. So occasionally, I would act regressively and babyish to get attention. Negative attention, but negative attention was better than none. I spent much of my childhood watching TV, playing "pretend" about being TV characters like

Flash Gordon, or hanging out in the backyard or the garage and doing mischief. As a 30-month-old left alone, I tried to examine a window fan. The stitches to repair my hand left marks that look like ancient runes:

> **Runes**
> When I was a toddler,
> Two and a half or so,
> I learned about a room fan,
> As children forgotten tend to do
> When left on their own.
> Sixty–seven stitches later
> The back of my left hand
> Has been inscribed with pale runes,
> Glyphs by which I guide my life.
> Deciphered:
> Do not need,
> Do not want,
> Do not love too well,
> And you will not be wounded.

I learned to hide in plain sight. When I got older, I would learn to disappear, hanging out at the library. I became extremely introverted and had no friends. I expected nothing and wouldn't have known how to make my emotional wants and needs known had I been able to identify them. I was never hugged and didn't know that I should have been.

I do not know what path I would have taken had I stayed in Los Angeles with my parents, because for high school, my parents sent me across the country to a boarding school near my aunt. At 14 I had to transform myself from a regressive, immature child, into a super independent adolescent who had to handle everything on his own. I had to learn to be a survivor. At the same time, I was a socially awkward adolescent who was uncomfortable with others.

Adolescence is a time when we learn to be adults. But, because I was busy trying to survive, and had never learned how to forge normal, healthy relationships, I ended up confining myself to a world of loneliness and isolation. I was depressed but didn't know it. I had thought what I felt was the normal human condition. Because I did not know that there were alternatives, a world of relationships, a world of connectedness, a world of possibilities.

I spent the first years of High School feeling rootless. The school year in New York. The summers in Los Angeles, where I felt alone and friendless.

As a result, I have no real friend in my life from that period. I left High School in the middle of the senior year to go across the street from Yeshiva University High School to Yeshiva College, and inertia kept me there for four years, graduating in 1977 with a BA in Psychology. The last thing I wanted was to spend the next four years trying to get an advanced degree in Psychology to work in the world. I wanted to join the real world. I wanted to be an adult, without any idea as to what that entailed

From Lost Child to Lost Adult

I entered my adult life unequipped to handle the emotional challenges that life presents. I felt that I didn't fit in anywhere, was sad, confused. I sought refuge from the world in regressive and addictive behaviors. Ill equipped for adulthood, I tried in any case to be an adult, looking for a job, looking for a relationship, looking for a place that I could call home. I had no ideas how to do this and my early adult life was marked by many abrupt beginnings, moving from one possibility to another trying to find my place in life:

Beginnings
Part of me is enamored with new beginnings,
a collator of fledgling lives, which I try to join
into a jangling entity of conjunctive lines,
a cubist reality of a life.
Beginnings not of small chiselings
but of grand new directions,
dismissing smoothed crimps and folds,
for the unblemished,
and sending what was before clattering to the floor
with a disdainful sweep of an arm.

I say this because I am traveling to where I was born and left,
to return only now.
There is no better place to start a life again, I surmise,
than where you were born.
There I had a tiny blue wrist tag
(boy) Herskovitz. it said,
hardly even a name to limit my realms.
There I will ask for another tag of endless potentialities
and fold it over and around,
a chrysalis to be clutched to my heart.

And there, before the expanse of newborns,
I will recite all the names I have accumulated during my lives,
Each name forming a vaporous relic on the window of the nursery,
to then dissipate.
As these vestiges fade, I remain with but
the uncharted possibilities of the unnamed,
and I can walk out into a town in which no one knows me
and presume to start anew.

Through my brother-in-law who practiced Industrial Medicine, I discovered the field of Industrial Safety, and spent a year-and-a-half getting an MA in that field. I finished my degree in a field in which I was miserable. In September 1978 I started working for corporate America at Essex Chemical Corporation, even though I could not fit into corporate culture. After less than a year there I was told to look for another position. Thus, in the beginning of 1979 I began to search for a new job

I also was busy searching for love, needing love so desperately. But intimacy also meant a threat of abandonment. Fearing abandonment even more than the attraction of love, my relationships became a "dance of intimacy", pursuing love and then drawing back when the specter of abandonment reared its head.

Intimacy
I cannot contain your needs
when you are near me,
When you are close
I feel inadequate.
Distance yourself from me
and I can mold the remembrance
into a shape I can contain
and love.
When you are near
all I manage is to silence
the static that crackles in my mind,
Quietness not love.
Go from me
so that I can love you
The distance shelters me,
and allows me
my stealthed love

It is in the beginning of 1979 I was set up with my future spouse Pearl Steinmetz and we married three and a half months after meeting. Now, as a married man, I had to try to learn to love someone. I realized that I had never really experienced true love from my parents who had been traumatized by abandonment, and that I knew nothing of intimacy, nothing of love. My marriage was doomed to be loveless unless I learned to love.

<u>A Love Poem</u>
You say I don't love you
I love you no different than my parents
loved me.
Isn't that love?
Neither of us knows.
Love has no formula
That can be held to the light.
I have what I felt
When my parents cared for me,
as they could.
Is that love?
Or are they impaired
Am I impaired
So that what I grasped
was too full of holes
to be anything real.
You say I don't hug you.
I will hold you.
You say I don't care enough or care too much.
I will care more or less.
You say I shout
From now on I will whisper.
The problem isn't proving to you that I am able to love
But believing it myself.

I ended up taking a job with Pearl's father as an insurance broker for diamond dealers through Lloyd's of London. I was unhappy at that job as well. I began looking around for alternatives to my current existence. The answer I came up with – moving to Israel.

It had been Pearl's dream to live in Israel. I had promised her under the wedding canopy that we would someday live in Israel. Dissatisfied occupationally and socially where I was, I had nothing keeping me in America.

So, five-and-a-half years after we married, we moved to Israel with our two children. Once again, I was hoping to start a new life. But as I was still the same dysfunctional person and had dealt with none of my underlying problems, my new life in Israel was much like my life in America. After the initial euphoria of a new beginning in a new country, I was miserable once again.

By the time I was forty, I had lived in eight different cities in America, five different communities in Israel, had tried three different areas of study, two different professions, had eight different jobs, and had yet to find a place or a job that made me happy. I was married without true emotional intimacy. I was a father who didn't enjoy fatherhood. I was lost, and I was miserable and so, I went for counseling. In counseling, I found out I was a 2g. And I started to dig myself out of the hole that I was in.

The List: Journey to Healing

In the mid-90s I started to read everything I could about the psychopathology of being a child of a Holocaust survivor. In my internet surfing, I came across a lot of interesting information. In one of the sites that I visited in 1999, I found the following link:

"Shamash has a Second Generation (2nd-Gen) discussion group for children and grandchildren of Holocaust survivors on their website. Go to our links section and you'll find the Shamash link under NYSERNET: Holocaust Information gopher. Once you get there, go to their Community Center section where you will find a list of all their newsgroups and mailing lists to which you can subscribe. There are about 200 members in their Second Generation group."

I joined The List and stated corresponding with The List members. I don't remember any names or the issues we discussed. What I do remember is how emotionally affected I was by the discussions, and how I safe I felt discussing them. It was a secure place where I could discuss my emotional issues or problems, ones I had thought previously were mine alone. It turned out that a lot of the issues I was struggling with were the exact same issues discussed on The List. And I started to bring up all sorts of emotional problems I had as result of being a 2g in the hope that, if I could find the words, then perhaps I could be cured:

Ineffable
In the face of the ineffable
There can be no words, they say,
only silence.

But my life has been measured by decades of silence,
not mere kilometers.
So the crunch of flagstones,
the swirl of winds,
even the tears
are no stead.
Here in Auschwitz silence will not suffice,
for when words return,
they return as they were,
like seeds scattered on the frozen ground.
But if a voice can rise from the desolation,
to parse therewith a syntax of the pain.
then words entombed shall resurgent flow,
words whose tears may heal the soul again

The more I wrote, the more I connected to The List members, the more I found that the ideas would come to me in verse, and that the emotions would be best expressed in poetry. I would spend my night online reading and responding, and then, early in the morning, the emotions would come into my head as poetry. I had a narrative to present to the world, and people wanted to listen. They said it was good. To me it didn't matter, I had things hidden deep inside that I had to say, and I believed if I said them, then perhaps I could heal:

<u>Emotions</u>
I allowed myself no emotion in the shadow of Auschwitz.
There was no room for my needs in a reality filled
With their hunger of then, their hunger of now.
In the shadow of Auschwitz I became dwarfed and unworthy.
So I burrowed any needs I had
It was better to not feel than to be shamed by my neediness,
Shredding the fabric of reality to build a nest of denial,
concealing my feelings beneath,
Muffling my cries.
But today I quarry to free them,
For a need can never be filled unless it is voiced,
Nor a pain allayed before it is named.
So I clasp them to my heart in furrowed fists
Praying that when I might unclench.
They will wither.

My poetry became a way for my inner child to voice his feelings, thoughts, and emotions. Perhaps I was looking for a way to connect to my parents, to say the words I should have said for decades. The distance that I feel is not so much one created from the geographical distance that has existed between us since high school, but an emotional distance between a child who never felt he was truly wanted or loved:

> **Out of Love**
> My mother fed me out of love.
> Out of love she clothed me,
> Tucking my shirttail in my pants.
> Out of love she first showed concern,
> then tried to transform,
> and when that failed she sent me away out of love
> so that elsewhere I might grow.
> Once away I would never return to her
> For a while she acted out of love,
> I have never felt within her love.
> And since I have known but amplitudes of love,
> Weaving in and out of intimacy,
> Cresting up then down,
> Turning back then away

As a Second Generation, I am uncomfortable expressing these feelings because they are an indictment of my parents. They have suffered too much pain, and it is not their fault that the Holocaust destroyed something within them. And I regret that. But these feelings burn within me, and I know they existed then because they exist in me now in my most intimate relationships. If I feel at times that I am incapable of love, it is because I was unable to feel their love as a child.

There is too much pain and guardedness in me. But if, via poetry, I am able to confront the pain, then healing is possible. The List provided me with a safe place to confront my feelings. By allowing me a safe place in which to vent my frustration and anger, The List allowed me the cathartic experience I required to process and resolve the problematics of my childhood. The creative process provided the distance needed from the Survivor parent, and the members of The List provided the support and acceptance of these feelings. Thus, I was able to go beyond my fear and anger to perceive the positive aspects of my upbringing, and the warmth that was expressed in peculiar ways:

Farewells

I went to say goodbye to my parents
when they left the country.
My mother was busy the entire visit
packing up the leftovers
so I hardly had a chance to say goodbye.
"Hurry home before the dairy products spoil"
was the last thing she said as she closed the door.
I stood in the parking lot
laden with Tupperware,
feeling alone.
The next day I sat hunched over her reheated soup,
my hands encircled the bowl,
warming my fingers,
steam rising about my face,
as I waited for the soup to cool.
It has taken too much of a lifetime
to learn to live in a family
where you eat soup
instead of saying goodbye.

The process of catharsis, dialogue, and reconciliation that was started on The List provided me a path to healing that has continued since. A hope that someday in the future, when I am older, I will be healed:

When I Get Older

When I get older
I will start to try to remember
What my mother has chosen to forget.
But in the meantime
leave me to glean fragments of words and glances
and set them aside.
When I get older
I will start to build a legacy
out of the grey mists of the past.
But in the meantime
leave me commemorations
of disconcerting silence
When I get older
I will buy pages gilded in gold
to write long and straight across ivory tint

> But in the meantime
> leave me my fortuitous scraps
>> on which to scrawl jagged sentences
>> that bend around stains and scribbles
> When I get older,
> I can start to imagine being someone
> I hadn't imagined before
> But in the meantime
> leave me to sit on the park bench ,
> between my parents,
> eating sandwiches out of waxed paper bags.

A person's world view can be changed. I had viewed the world as a survivor, a world fraught with dangers to be avoided or and trials to be endured. A joyless place:

> <u>Wading</u>
> As I child I was taught
> That ours is an existence
> Of sadness and tears,
> Of anger and too few embraces,
> Of forgotten pasts and futures uncertain.
> I have since laid awake
> At nights remembering pasts
> I want to forget
> And at dawns previewing stumblings
> At obstacles yet encountered.
> I spend my days
> Wading in the ripples
> Casting about for moments of happiness
> Tinged with melancholy

As creativity enabled me to touch the traumatic memory, and to process it, my world view changed. Via poetry I was able to see the world as a place of possibility. That perhaps there was the potential to be blessed.

> <u>Curses and Blessings</u>
> At the bus stop he pointed at me in recognition
> But I showed no sign.
> Undaunted he came and shook my hand, his silver-framed glasses askew.
> "Let me finish my say then you can speak," he said

"May God bless you three blessings
That you join in the building of the third Temple,
That you live to see your children and grandchildren under the wedding canopy
That all your enemies be vanquished.
I am mentally ill,
Please give me some money so I can go to Yehezkel's grocery
And buy some food."
Which I did.
Some would dismiss this incident but I have not.
You see, my mother stood on the frozen muddied ground of Auschwitz,
Whose cursed soil petrified generations of lives
And I like to think that now God sends his peculiar messengers
to bless me,
And resuscitate my soul.

Slowly, my need for The List sort of disappeared, as it did for many others. Concurrently, we lost our home at Shamash, and moved en masse to Smartgroups. But the electricity wasn't there. We had been dealing with our problems long enough that The List became a litany of everyday life issues that really didn't justify having a List. When Smartgroups closed down, The List then moved to Yahoo groups, but it wasn't the same, and people just stopped posting as much. I started to read posts but never answered or posted myself. Maybe we grew up. Maybe we got tired. Maybe we stopped being so different and started to feel like everyone else.

This is the journey I made on The List between 1999 and 2004, in which poetry served as the vehicle for the journey, from silence, to dialogue, to healing. Poetry functions as a form of expression and protest, to communicate and to grieve, to vent and to comfort, and ultimately, it serves as an expression of change and hope.

The five years I spent on The List writing poetry blossomed into an education initiative called Creating.Memory. Because poetry gave me the words in which to express my inner world, I felt that it could also help future generations connect to the Holocaust and thus, in 2019, I started a project which asks students to explore, via the creative process, key themes present in the Holocaust and its aftermath, which are also relevant to today. The goal is to create a remembrance forged via creative expression, in which they have their own unique voice.

Using the creative process, Creating.Memory enables an emotional language that has never been used by survivors and their children, theologians and historians, to process the trauma. A language that enables expression of latent pain and the working through of the traumatic memory. Uriel Nativ, a playback theater instructor who conducted a Creating.Memory workshop for high school students, commented on the experience:

"It appears that, even with the most difficult materials, it is possible to create. Some of the guys came to the workshop, as expected, more than a little wary of the workshop – "Shoah again?" And then, slowly, the understanding that this time, something else is happening…. Instead of the same old texts' rote commemorations, you encounter an experience that is relevant to your life, related to one's own world, but a little different. Suddenly, you are creating on your own. You are letting these materials resonate within you, and from inside you to others. The encounter with the memory in this way gave me, and them, freedom to touch these matters freely and honestly, via a vivid creative experience. And the memory becomes meaningful, varied, rich and full of emotion."

I will be forever grateful to The List for the opportunity to plumb my emotional depths, for the support afforded me there, and for the role it had in making me the person I am today.

Clara Jacob
You've Got 2G Mail

The most important event in my life happened before I was born.
I don't remember where I read this, but I understood it instantly and have never forgotten those words. The event, of course, was the Holocaust. I grew up knowing very little about it and even less about my father's Holocaust experience. And I was completely unaware of its influence on me and my family.

I didn't know anyone else (except my father's two sisters) who had any relationship to the Holocaust. I didn't even know any Jewish people. When I finally met Jews, in college, I assumed we would have an instant bond because of the Holocaust. I couldn't have been more wrong.

It wasn't until my mid-30s that I began to glimpse its impact on me.

First, I met the man I would eventually marry. He was Lakota, and when I told him about my background, he said, "So you understand genocide." It was the first time anyone had recognized and valued that part of me. Second, my father decided at age 70 that he wanted to tell his story. He, my mom, my brother, and I went to Paris to see where he had lived as a child, gone to school, and hidden from the Nazis. Third, I found a group of people online who were also children of Holocaust survivors. And even though they were complete strangers, these people understood me, deeply and profoundly.

The Family Twig

Like most people, I have two family trees – my mother's and my father's. The tree on my mother's side is like a Redwood, immense and firmly rooted. It includes English lords with castles in the 1300s, a Chief Justice of the United States Supreme Court, and a Captain George Denison, who arrived in New England in 1631; his home in Mystic, Connecticut, is now a museum.

The tree on my father's side is more like a twig. My father Bernard, and his two younger sisters, were born in Paris. Their parents were Romanian Jewish immigrants who had met in Paris as young adults. Bernard's father, Paul, for whom my brother was named, was from Bucharest. That's all that my father ever learned about his father's family or history. Bernard's mother, Therese, came from a small village in Romania. Her maiden name was Abase and she had three aunts in Paris (her mother, Clara, for who I was named, stayed in Romania). The aunts were named Henriette, Mathilde, and Pauline. And that's all my father ever learned about his mother's family or history.

My grandparents fled Romania because of increasing antisemitism. I suspect that my grandfather's experiences were so traumatic that he wouldn't, or couldn't, share them.

Truly, it is a privilege to have a family tree.

Born in 1930, Bernard was 4 years older than Ginette, and 10 years older than Mimi. The family was poor, isolated, and assimilated; they socialized mostly with the great aunts. Paul and Therese spoke Yiddish, Romanian, and French at home. On High Holy Days, Bernard and his father went to *shul* (synagogue). As a young boy, Bernard felt very much loved by his mother, and felt safe until the Germans occupied Paris.

In 1942, the Germans required Jews to register and wear stars. Bernard wasn't happy with how his father, a tailor, sewed the yellow star onto his jacket. The edges weren't flat, so his father fixed it for him. Later he felt immense regret and guilt about that. He still has the star to this day.

"Rumors about mass roundups of Jews began to circulate and those who could afford it fled," Bernard wrote. "Somehow, my parents learned that aunts Henriette and Mathilde intended to leave Paris. My parents were very upset by that, and I remember us all going to see both aunts, and my parents begging them to let us come along and they turned us down. My parents and we, the children, felt quite dejected and depressed. We were completely on our own, and there was nowhere to go."

While Henriette and her son Georges escaped and survived the war, Mathilde and her daughter were robbed and killed by the man they'd hired to help them cross the border. Pauline survived the war and moved to Haifa, Israel.

The family went into hiding in a small town outside Paris, Vigneux-sur-Seine. Paul took the train to the city to work and returned in the evening; the family would wait for him at the train station. Bernard would sometimes take a later morning train to Paris and then the subway to "work" with his father. On September 24, 1942, Bernard did just that, and discovered when he arrived that the police had taken his father. The concierge, who had handed him over to the police, told Bernard to go to the police station.

"I ran to the police station and my father was there, waiting for me. He was very happy to see me...He said I should go back to Vigneux and tell my mother, and help her take care of the girls," Bernard wrote. They sat together on a bench. "As we had said our goodbyes, both in tears, my father said to the policeman, 'The boy can go, can't he?' The policeman looked at me and looked at my father and said, 'Why do you put yourself in the lion's mouth?' My father said, 'GO NOW!' and I ran out." Bernard returned to Vigneux, but Paul Jacob never returned, and no one heard from him ever again. Later Bernard found his name on a list of deportees to Auschwitz.

In Vigneux, Therese worked as a domestic for a well-known doctor who was prominent in the French underground. When police raided his home on January 14, 1943, they found her, and turned her over to the Germans. Bernard received several postcards from his mother, sent from Drancy. She assured him everything was all well, and told Bernard to look after Ginette, then age 9 and Mimi, who was 2. Much later, Bernard found her name, too, on a list of those transported to Auschwitz.

The Jacob children were in contact with an organization that helped Jewish orphans. They were taken back to Paris to stay temporarily, receiving new Christian names. Eventually a group of 10 or 12 of these children, chaperoned by several young adults, rode a train to the Swiss border, posing as young campers with camp counselors and illegally crossing the border. In Switzerland, the siblings were split up. Cute little Mimi went to a loving home. Ginette lucked out with a wealthy family who adored her. Bernard was a rightfully angry teenager, shuttled from one foster home to another. His final placement was with a pair of elderly sisters just across the border from Germany, who doted on him.

After the war, Ginette and Mimi were sent to an orphanage in Paris while Bernard stayed in Switzerland. An American family adopted Mimi and soon sponsored Bernard to come to the United States. He moved to New York City, and got a job as a courier at a small publishing company. The secretary, Rosamond Tryon, was tasked with taking him to lunch on his first day. That turned out to be my parents' first date.

Nobody in Rosamond's WASPy family approved of her marrying a penniless, orphaned Jewish immigrant who didn't speak English, but she did so anyway. She was 21 and Bernard was just 19. Bernard brought Ginette to the United States and she lived with my parents for six years until she finished college and medical school.

Bernard and Rosamond enjoyed the artistic and literary riches of New York. Eventually they moved to Rosamond's hometown, Minneapolis, Minnesota, where Bernard finished his studies to become an architect. And on September 30, 1958, they welcomed to the world a baby girl who they named Clara.

The Second Generation

As Bernard and Rosamond's first child, I was well-loved. My earliest memory is the day my younger brother was born, a few months before my third birthday. We lived in St. Paul, Minnesota, in an old house in a middle-class, heavily Roman Catholic neighborhood. As a young child, I was shy, stubborn, and smart (mostly still true). Already at age 4, I remember feeling that my family was unlike other families.

My father had a foreign accent. He wore knee socks with shorts. We ate food that was weird (such as quiche) and stinky (garlic). Every child I knew ate Oscar Meyer bologna sandwiches with mayonnaise on Wonder Bread while watching TV. My parents called Wonder Bread "bath-towel bread" and purchased exotic rye from a local bakery. We listened to classical music, loved and accumulated books, went to art museums, and watched our black-and-white TV so rarely that we would take it out when we wanted to use it, and put it away when a show ended.

Other children talked about God and Jesus. I didn't know who God and Jesus were, and was ostracized one summer because of that. I had dark hair and a darker complexion than most kids in our neighborhood and was forever being asked, "What *are* you?"

I remember clearly when I first learned of the Holocaust. My mother told me what had happened to my grandparents. How they were treated like animals and tricked into taking a "shower" that killed them. It shook me to the core to learn that people could be so cruel. I cried and cried. My mother comforted me and asked why I was crying. I said I felt sad for my father because his parents were dead. She told me, "Oh, he's fine, it happened a long time ago, and he's over it." Much later I understood just how untrue this statement was.

My family was not Jewish – but we were not exactly Christian, either. We joined a Unitarian Universalist (UU) church, possibly for the optics, which at the time was a hotbed of hippies. My parents were atheists, but the path of least resistance was being culturally Christian to accommodate my mother's family. We had a Christmas tree, sang carols, and exchanged presents, but nobody even pretended to believe in what we celebrated.

My father liked going to midnight Mass on Christmas, for the music, art, and ritual. When we were a little older, he admitted that he was sort of a fan of Catholics, who had welcomed him when his family was hiding outside of Paris. He definitely had not felt welcomed by Lutherans in Switzerland, and when he went to a synagogue in St. Paul one evening, he was stopped at the door by men demanding to know who he was, which was so unwelcoming that he turned around and left.

We did not live near either of my father's sisters. Aunt Ginette was married to Uncle Josh and my cousins, two girls, were a few years younger than I was. They lived in New York. Aunt Mimi visited us once, and we visited her several times in Chicago. When she got married, we attended her beautiful and lavish wedding in Grand Rapids, Michigan. This was the first time I had been to any type of Jewish gathering, or seen any man wearing a yarmulke. I had to wear a pink dress with ankle socks and patent leather shoes, and I remember hating everything about the outfit.

My brother and I were sent to the children's table. When an older girl asked who we were, I said Mimi was our aunt. The girl said, "No she isn't, she's OUR aunt and we don't know you!" I had been told that Mimi had an adopted family, but apparently that family didn't know about us. It was like we were a secret family. Aside from that awkwardness, the event was magical – endless food, women in glamorous formal dresses, live music, dancing, and a wonderful moment when the groom stamped on a glass and a great cry went up among the guests.

Our family did not talk about the Holocaust. During my childhood, a documentary was released featuring footage from the liberation of the concentration camps. My mother mentioned that she and my father watched the program and it had upset him. She looked worried and sad. My father never told me and my brother about his past directly, so all our information came from my mother. Over the years, she would share a bit more, so we had a rough idea of what had happened to him. But it was treated like a secret. And so, it felt like a secret. And when kids said, "What *are* you?" I felt like there was a secret to protect – a secret I needed to hide.

Our neighborhood and the nearby schools were very homogenous. For the most part, everyone was white and Christian. The elementary school I attended was a few blocks from home. I was one of the younger students in my grade, and I often felt at a disadvantage socially.

In first grade I didn't color within the lines in my *Dick and Jane* coloring book, so I was made to sit out in the hall as a punishment, and a second grader was sent to teach me how to color. Of course, I knew how to color perfectly well, but in our home, I wasn't allowed to use coloring books because art and creativity were prized.

My skill in academics, and complete lack of skill in athletics, were evident by third and fourth grade. I got good grades without trying very hard and in math class especially, I found my imagination far more interesting than the teacher's lessons. The last concept in math I really understood was long division; after that, it was all a mystery because I'd stopped paying attention. But reading and writing came naturally to me.

In fourth grade, our all-white school was integrated by school busing. This meant that children of color – Black, Native and Mexican-American – were taken from their own neighborhood schools and their friends, and brought to our school. These kids looked the way I often felt – miserable, alone, and out of place. They'd rush to the bus when school was dismissed so as not to miss the ride home. More than once, children I'd gone to school with since kindergarten thought I was one of the children who rode the bus and would helpfully let me know the bus was about to leave.

I enjoyed fifth and sixth grade, for the most part. It was fun to be among the older children in the school, to have the responsibility of being part of safety patrol, and to have a tiny bit more freedom during the day. During lunchtime a friend and I would sometimes go to her house and watch a soap opera on TV, something I would never be allowed to do at home.

In addition to feeling like I didn't belong, I was often angry. One of my earliest memories is of being in a playpen, wanting to get out, and being furious that I couldn't. As I grew older, I continued to be angry. It often felt like outrage over injustice. Growing up in the 1960s, I was exposed to the civil rights movement. My mother took me to peace marches and women's rights rallies. I remember walking at night in the rain through the city streets as part of an enormous protest after Dr. Martin Luther King, Jr. was shot and killed. It was OK to be angry about discrimination. When an older neighborhood kid said the N-word in my backyard, I punched him, and he ran home.

At times, my anger seemed to erupt from nowhere. I was the only one in the family who would stamp, yell, and express anger. I didn't understand why I was so mad. My brother was easier to deal with, and I felt my parents liked him better. My feelings intensified as I became a teenager. I was continuously at odds with my father. I was selfish, mildly disobedient, and no doubt unpleasant to be around. But my approximately 13-year-long adolescence wasn't easy on me, either. My emotions were all-consuming. One minute I would be raging, the next crying, and the next completely numb. It was exhausting.

When I turned 15, I was finally able to get a job, which gave me a little more control over my life. My parents wouldn't let me talk on the phone for more than 10 minutes, so with my earnings, I got my own phone line and rotary dial phone with a cord long enough to reach into my room. My first job was scooping ice cream at Baskin-Robbins; the uniform for the all-girl crew was short pink polyester dresses with pantyhose. But handing ice cream cones to smiling customers was one of my better employment experiences.

I went to a large public high school, against my father's wishes; he preferred a private prep school that my younger brother ended up attending. At St. Paul Central, I was invited to join an alternative learning program within the school, designed for highly motivated students. We had special classes and created our own independent study courses, complete with learning contracts and evaluations. I got credit for studying poetry, learning to take, develop and print photos, working in the county attorney's office, working in a social service agency serving troubled youth, and skydiving. I'm still amazed that I was allowed to graduate without taking any math, science, or social studies courses during my junior and senior years.

After graduating from high school, I went to Vassar College, which was two hours north of New York City and more than 1,200 miles from home. As a Midwesterner surrounded by wealthy New Yorkers, I was very much out of my element. And as a socially awkward introvert, I was excruciatingly uncomfortable almost everywhere. Most of my classmates had attended exclusive prep schools, while at my public high school with its alternative program, I hadn't even learned how to structure an essay.

College was also the first time I met Jewish people outside of my own family. I was so excited to become friends with them! I anticipated that we would instantly connect, and I would be welcomed into their world – and that my Holocaust connection would be a sort of badge of honor.

I didn't lead with the fact that my grandparents died in Auschwitz but found a time to share that fact fairly quickly after learning that someone was Jewish. Imagine my dismay when one Jewish person after another had absolutely no interest in the topic! In fact, I received disdainful looks, and later they would try to avoid me.

Finally, a kind Jewish guy clued me in, explaining that the Holocaust wasn't something that American Jews typically bonded over. It was not badge of honor, but a source of shame because it meant one's family wasn't rich or connected enough to have escaped. Also, nobody wanted to talk about the Holocaust; it was horrible, and it was history. Again, my family background was something to keep secret.

My academic experience at college was excellent. I majored in English with a creative writing concentration. In retrospect, I believe I was depressed during college. I also started developing migraines. After college, I lived in New York for five years. There, for the first time, my physical appearance was completely normal; nobody ever asked, "What *are* you?" Overall, I was fairly self-destructive but came to my senses after having a beautiful baby girl, Iris, and running away from her abusive father, back to Minneapolis. After a lot of therapy, I found a better path that led to an exceptional career opportunity in Sioux Falls, South Dakota.

I often wonder why I thought moving to South Dakota was a good idea, but for a single mother struggling to earn enough to be comfortable, it was a solution. Also, Iris's father had come to Minneapolis looking for us, but I knew he'd never come to South Dakota. My nightmares about him stopped and I began to feel that I could move about freely.

Although it was safe, I was acutely aware that we were out of place in such a rural area. Iris was Black and I was a single mother who looked Native; we knew no one in the area, and it was as though people had never seen a Black person or a multi-racial family. They asked ridiculous questions, made sweeping assumptions, and were often downright racist. It was difficult, and I still regret subjecting Iris to that environment.

While working full time, I completed a long-distance MFA in creative writing program. In 1993, I met Mike, an Oglala Lakota man from the Pine Ridge Reservation. During one of our early phone calls, he asked, "What *are* you?" and like many others who had asked me that question, he thought I was Native American. I told him my "secret", and the magic words that made sparks fly for me were, "So you understand genocide."

He had long hair, which I always liked on men. His intelligence matched mine, and his life story was extraordinary; in fact, we got to know each other because he asked me to write his biography. We loved to talk about ideas. The magic words that made sparks fly for him were, "It has been proven that there is no scientific, physical reason for the past to exist prior to the future."

My parents were not exactly thrilled by my decision to marry Mike, just as my mother's parents hadn't been thrilled with her choice. I had fallen in love with a man from the poorest county in the United States, where the average life expectancy for a man was 49 and where the unemployment rate is 90 %.

We married in 1994, and had two children, Mica and Mato (which means bear in Lakota). Mike was a social worker who helped Lakota people, and in graduate school, he began reading about intergenerational trauma and shared this information with me. I couldn't help but notice that most of the large-scale studies cited focused not on Indigenous people, but on Holocaust survivors.

In 2000, my dad turned 70. To celebrate his birthday, he wanted to take me, my mother, and my brother to Paris, to see where he grew up. He said that he didn't want to be like his father, who had not shared anything about his past. My dad was ready to tell his story. We traveled to Paris and packed a lot of walking and talking into a few days' time. We saw where my dad grew up; the apartment building was gone, another was in its place, but we walked around the neighborhood, saw where he had attended school, where he had walked with his parents, where he had played. On another day we went to the village where the family went into hiding.

Walking from one place to another one day, we stumbled upon a synagogue that looked familiar to my dad. Once inside, he remembered going there with his father. We even went to a cemetery on the outskirts of Paris and found the graves of Aunt Henriette and her family. During the entire trip, my brother videotaped our journey and my father's words.

The information we learned from my father in Paris was golden, but it was intense and emotional. Back home, I felt sorrow and hopelessness, as though I had somehow absorbed all the pain – not just my father's, but the pain of his mother and his father – and had to carry this burden.

I searched for information online. If there were studies of survivors, maybe someone knew what their children went through, which might be related to what I was feeling. At the time, I thought the term "survivor" only applied to concentration camp survivors (and so did my father). I thought there must be a reading list or an association or support group that could help me sort through my feelings.

Joining the List

I don't recall exactly how I found "The List," but I believe I had to "apply." It was extremely intimidating. Since I didn't yet believe that I was a second generation (2g) survivor, I felt like I was an imposter, trying to gain access to the group through falsely claiming to be a 2g. Still, somehow, I was drawn to become a member. I hadn't been able to fully process the trip to Paris; it was as though it were stuck in my throat, impossible to dislodge.

It was 2000 or 2001. We had just returned to Sioux Falls from St. Louis, Missouri, where we'd lived while my husband completed his master's degree. I didn't particularly want to live in Sioux Falls, but it was halfway between Mike's parents and my parents (a four-hour drive, in opposite directions). We were the oldest children in our respective families and felt a responsibility to them. Finally, I received word that I was allowed to join The List.

At the time, The List was very active. When I started reading, I felt like someone had turned on a firehose. Multiple discussion threads were happening at once, and dozens of participants were simultaneously sharing, commenting, commiserating and arguing. Conversation was lively, vigorous, and often contentious.

I hadn't known what to expect, but I thought The List would be more like a support group than a boxing ring. I'd imagined I would write about my deep sorrow and kind group members would console me and share their own, very similar personal experiences. Instead, I struggled to understand what List members were even talking about. This began with basic vocabulary. What was *tsuris*? *Daven*? *Kvell*? *Tallis*? *Chuppah*? What was *Yahrzeit*? *Sukkot*? *Mikveh*? Did all the women wear wigs? Why did people clean obsessively before *Pesach* (and what was *Pesach*, anyway?)? Why were people so angry about inconsequential things?

During my first months on The List, I shared very little. I could barely keep up with the barrage of daily emails, what with working full time and three children. I tried to piece together who was who – the fact that there were several sets of women with the same name made it more complicated. And why were there 2gs living in Australia? China? South America?

Early on, I learned that my father was definitely a survivor, which made me an authentic 2g. At least I belonged in that sense, which I desperately wanted. Then again, I didn't belong. I discovered that virtually everyone on The List was Jewish. This should not have been surprising, but once again I felt like I didn't fit in. On The List I soon found that according to some rules, if my mother wasn't a Jew, I couldn't be Jewish at all. According to other rules, my father wasn't even Jewish since he didn't participate in Jewish life. Was Judaism a religion? A race? A culture?

When I posed questions or chimed in, I would receive some helpful comments. Most List members didn't seem to feel as isolated or unaccountably angry and sad in the way I did. But we all shared the experience of having parents whose lives overshadowed our own. Some List members' parents were liberated from concentration camps. Others were in hiding throughout the war. Some were in the resistance. More than a few of the parents already had a spouse and children who they'd lost. And others married fellow survivors after meeting in a Displaced Persons Camp.

It seemed that Holocaust survivor parents either didn't talk at all about what happened to them or talked about nothing else. From what I could tell, many of the parents had severe mental health issues stemming from PTSD. In other words – I thought my family was crazy, but some of the families described were next level crazy. The survivors were damaged in dozens of different ways, all of which made complete sense. Their behaviors ranged from extreme anxiety to debilitating depression and everything in between. List members described what to me sounded like horrific abuse at the hands of the very people who cherished them beyond belief. Then again, I witnessed intense anger and disagreements between List members, sometimes resulting in a member leaving for a while or for good.

I felt fortunate that I'd experienced a relatively mild "case" of survivor behavior. Of course, we're all more comfortable with our own family's dysfunctions than other families' dysfunction. However, most of The List members had something I didn't – a community. Some List members had families that regularly socialized with other survivor families. Most families were also part of a community of Jews, whether formal or informal. To me, having a historical or cultural link would have been worth all the family dysfunction in the world.

Still hungry for clues about my own life, I ordered and devoured books that List members recommended. I didn't have to look far to find myself in those pages. It was comforting to finally understand what was "wrong with me." Themes like sorrow, anger, guilt, shame, secrecy, blame, lateral violence, and identity were common. Isolation was not mentioned as frequently.

During this time, Mike was again providing mental health services to Lakota people, and we made more frequent trips to Pine Ridge to visit his family and participate in cultural and spiritual activities. As I came to know List members' stories better, I saw parallels between the Lakota culture and the 2g experience. One of the similarities was the importance of family to both List members and my Lakota relatives. Everyone says family is the most important thing, but most people don't mean it. But I saw List member families and Lakota families actually living it.

Then there was the value of history, culture, and language. In a world that is fundamentally hostile to one's existence, much energy is spent on knowing one's history, participating in one's culture and mastering one's language. And an equal amount of energy is spent on protecting that history, culture, and language from those who want it destroyed – to the point where outsiders become unwelcome. Judaism and List members had no interest in recruiting converts, while the Lakota people would say, "We just want to be left alone." Another similarity was names. Many of the List members had Hebrew names, just as most of the Lakota people I knew had Lakota names (mine is *Wigmuke Hanska Win*, which means Long Rainbow Woman).

But much of what I saw in common was the result of trauma. Its effects were devastating, and when people were powerless to express their feelings outwardly, they often turned to self-destruction. Everyone was in pain.

Understanding this explained why some List members' parents seemed so cruel, just as it explained why some of my in-laws seemed so tortured.

My own mother-in-law, Delores, had been taken from her family and put into a Catholic residential school when she was four years old. The residential schools were the setting for appalling abuses of all kinds, including forbidding the children to speak their own language. Delores remembered her grandmother saying she had heard the sounds of the Wounded Knee Massacre in 1890 from a nearby school.

As damaged as they were by one misguided and genocidal government policy after another, the Lakota people were very much alive. I witnessed the connection between the people and the power of their culture, language, and a shared history.

I struggled to fit in both on The List and in my husband's family. Existing on the periphery of the Jewish world and the Lakota world, I was part of both, yet part of neither. However, despite what I wasn't, I was still a person who was angry about injustice. Through my involvement in anti-racist organizations, I became friends with a wonderful woman who turned out to be Jewish. Sara invited me to the local congregation, Mount Zion Temple, to visit. I was very excited to participate! I attended with Sara several times. She introduced me to the very small group of people, who were friendly, and explained to me what was happening during services.

Unfortunately, I was disappointed. I had expected a magical experience – that my soul would recognize an ancestral connection and I would be transported into a sacred realm. Instead, what I found was that a Jewish service was very similar to a Christian service. We were all sitting in rows, while people talked to us from the front of the room, and not only did we use a book, but it was apparently the SAME book, minus the fluffy new section. I felt the same as I felt after any Christian service, which was nothing.

Part of my reaction stemmed from being involved in Lakota spiritual practices. The equivalent of attending services was participating in an *inipi*, or sweat lodge ceremony. We sat in a circle on the ground inside a small, round, tent-like structure covered with tarps and blankets, through which no light could penetrate. Rocks heated by fire for several hours were ritually placed in the center of the *inipi*. Water was poured on the rocks as we sang specific Lakota songs, prayed and smoked the *cannupa*, or pipe, over the course of several hours. There were other ceremonies I took part in, as well, such as the *Wiwang Waci,* or sun dance, which were even more unusual. From a Lakota perspective, Judaism and Christianity really were relatively similar.

On The List, I mentioned attending Jewish services and being disappointed. List members encouraged me to continue participating and to learn more about Judaism, since I didn't fully understand what was happening. Fair enough, I thought. I learned that Mount Zion's visiting student rabbi (there weren't enough people in the congregation for a full-time rabbi) would be leading a 16-week Introduction to Judaism class and together with Sara, I signed up.

When the class first met, I was shocked that about half of the congregation had also signed up for the class. Did these folks not know about their own religion? I asked Sara why she was attending, and she said that she wanted a refresher.

It was a surprisingly rigorous course. We were assigned a great deal of reading, and each class was three to four hours long. It didn't take long for me to understand why one would need a refresher. There was an enormous quantity of information, wisdom, and scholarship, including nearly 6,000 years of history.

After the first few classes, I pulled back a bit from participating in The List. Despite having always been welcomed, I felt that I had no right to represent myself as even a little bit Jewish. In my course, we were barely scratching the surface, yet I had glimpsed the vastness and complexity of Judaism – enough to know what I did not and would never know.

Yet, The List became a place of refuge for me, and still the only place I could share certain parts of myself. When I saw that I had 2g mail, I would generally drop whatever I was doing and read the latest List message. With the many conversations on every topic under the sun happening simultaneously, The List was for me a social group and therapy group rolled into one and truly a more consistent presence than most of my friends or family.

Into the Wild

One of the fun aspects of The List was hearing about members meeting up outside the formal group structure. For instance, if an American List member was traveling to Israel, he or she would get together with Israeli List members and New York List members would gather from time to time. Even though I was not part of any of these events, stranded as I was in the Midwest, I enjoyed them vicariously.

I must have written on The List that I wished that I could meet group members. Someone suggested I attend an upcoming 2g (Second Generation) conference in Chicago. I wasn't sure what people would be conferring about, but I decided to try it out. Predictably, it was cold and windy in

Chicago, but warm, in every sense, inside the conference hotel. I realized that there was a sort of survivor/2g conference circuit, with speakers, entertainers and attendees who traveled from one to the next. Many of the participants already knew each other and moved around in groups.

It was great fun to meet List members and put faces to names! I felt strange about meeting someone for the first time when we already knew intimate details about each other's lives. I had seen a few photos of selected List members, but for the most part I had absolutely no idea what they looked like or sounded like until meeting them. I remember a few List members being surprised by my voice – my flat Midwestern accent and demeanor turned people off, as it had when I was in college. I was shocked to overhear a conversation among a group of women that began with the question: "Have you ever been inside a church?" Most of the women had never been in a church, which amazed me and underlined the fact that the world I came from was completely different from theirs.

Aside from the more serious sessions, the conference seemed to be mostly an opportunity to socialize. I connected rather deeply with some List members. Two of my favorite memories from that event seemed to fit together. One evening I got a huge hug from Fivel, the son of a List member, that almost made me cry. The next day, another List member and I braved sub-zero hurricane-force winds to visit the Spertus Institute. There, in a large Klarsfeld book listing the names of French Holocaust victims, I found my grandparents listed, just as my father had, many years before. But instead of being named Therese and Paul, they were Tauba and Pavel. As my List friend noted, I had found MY Fivel.

Most of the conferences for 2gs were co-sponsored by Survivor organizations. Back home, I was encouraged by List members to attend another conference and bring my father. It was not an easy sell. During my childhood, my father dealt with matters of the Holocaust through avoidance. Then, in Paris, he told us his story. I imagine he felt that his job was done. I knew that if I could convince my mother to attend the upcoming conference, chances were good that she would persuade him.

My mother succeeded, and the three of us went to Toronto. Immediately, I felt my father's discomfort. I came across a few List members at the conference, but during most meals or full group sessions I would sit with my parents. During one dinner, when everyone was eating together in a large room, a shouting match broke out. My mother became afraid and wanted to leave the room. My father was slightly amused. I was not at all surprised, based on how I'd seen people behave on The List.

The sessions were good, but the information was beginning to feel repetitive. My father looked overwhelmed most of the time, and my mother worked hard to take care of him and his feelings, which was normal. At dinner one night, my father said he'd visited with a woman who knew of or had been involved with an organization that helped the orphaned Jewish children in Switzerland. After the war, people from the organization traveled around Switzerland to find the children and bring them into the fold, so to speak, helping them to reconnect with their communities and culture, and in some cases, relocate. She asked my father if he'd had a bar mitzvah. My father said he hadn't, and that that nobody had come to find him. The woman expressed her condolences. "We must have missed you," she said.

After the conference, I went back to my home in South Dakota and my parents returned to Minneapolis. A few weeks later my mother told me that my father had been extremely depressed and had resolved to never again attend anything like the conference. Of course, this left me feeling guilty for subjecting him to so much pain.

Inspired by the conference, I decided to capture my family's story. I went to New York and did audio interviews with Aunt Ginette and Aunt Mimi to capture their memories. I spent much time preparing to do the interviews properly, learning how oral history is gathered and finding tips specifically for interviewing survivors. Aunt Ginette's story was very non-linear, and it differed from my father's story on some important points. She did have a photo album with pictures I'd never seen. Aunt Mimi didn't remember anything about France or Switzerland.

Next, I digitized the videotapes my brother had made. It turned out to be 16 hours of footage. I had intended to match the audio interviews up with the video, but it was a daunting task. The more I watched, the more painful it became, and nobody in the family seemed interested in the project or the end result. I couldn't proceed. I copied the footage and interviews onto flash drives and sent them to any family member who wanted one.

By then, I'd also begun to cringe when the Holocaust came up. My husband and I realized that we both had a sort of historical trauma fatigue. If my book club read a book about the Holocaust, I skipped it. If an award-winning film involving the Holocaust came out, I did not want to see it. It was simply too painful. Similarly, when TV shows about Lakota history or the Wounded Knee Massacre or even Westerns came on, my husband did not want to watch. He already knew the story, and watching it just created pain.

My mother died in 2015 at 87, and my husband died in 2020, at age 61 (beating the 49-year-old life expectancy by a few years, but still much too young). Aunt Ginette died in 2021. At age 91, my father is physically and cognitively healthy. Recently we were guests at another large Jewish wedding in Michigan; my brother Paul's son, Nick, married a beautiful and accomplished woman in 2018. Jordan comes from a large, tightknit Jewish family, and Nick happily converted to Judaism. They are expecting their first child in early 2022, who will be my father's fourth great-grandchild – another 4g.

I can't help but think of my grandparents, Pavel and Tauba. I imagine the hopes and dreams they had for their own lives and their children's lives. I think about how they felt being taken away from their small family; their fear and despair, and how anguished they must have been about their children. It's trite to say they would be proud of their children, grandchildren, great-grandchildren, and great-great-grandchildren, but they would be. They would scoff at guilt and identity issues – we should just be thankful to be among the living. I think they would also be astonished by all the life they set in motion, that grew and flourished despite the best efforts of the Nazis.

Just as Holocaust survivors are becoming old and passing away, List members too are aging. It's now up to us to tell our parents' stories. I don't interact much, and I still avoid Holocaust and 2g subject matter. But The List remains important to me, and as long as I see that I've got 2g mail, I'll be there.

Gail Ellen Rubinstein Lipton
My Journey – Discovery, Connection, and Community

Introduction

As a naïve 16-year-old, I spent the summer before my Senior year as a foreign exchange student in Doxato, Greece, a small, isolated town near the Bulgarian border. I thought it would be similar to the small hamlet on Long Island where I grew up, and I wasn't worried at all. I had never experienced antisemitism. I had also never been away from home for more than a week at a time, and only to Girl Scout camp (which I hated). I didn't speak Greek, but thought I'd be able to pick it up easily since I had an aptitude for languages, could read the Greek alphabet, and carried a mini dictionary with me.

I wanted to get away, but I had no idea what I was walking into. I was unaware that the entire Jewish community in northern Greece had been exterminated thirty years earlier, and that the one synagogue in the bordering town was locked up. I never dreamed that people wouldn't know what a Jew looked like – but they kept looking for my horns and asking why I didn't have a large nose. There was no malice – they hadn't seen a Jew in thirty years, and they were curious. Since no one in the town spoke any English, in my broken Greek I tried to answer their questions as best I could.

I spent several months in Greece, and then returned to my comfortable life as a high school student in Carle Place. I believe I was more sensitive to things going on around me than before I left. I considered myself to be the child of a survivor, but my dad had passed away several months before I left, so he was no longer around to talk to.

Fast forward several decades. I left Carle Place to attend college in Philadelphia, and after two decades living and working there, I moved with my family to Maryland. Besides my full-time job, I became a principal and teacher in several religious schools. As a Jewish educator I felt compelled to ensure that students could identify with their heritage, begin to trace their family history, and have at least some basic knowledge of the Shoah. The most meaningful way to educate them was by using first-person experiences and second-generation knowledge. I harnessed my energy into researching as much as I could about my own family to pique their interest, show them how to obtain information, and bring them closer to history. It was during my research that my cousin introduced me to The List.

To me the 2g (Second Generation) List is not just a way to hear about others' family experiences before, during, and after the war. It is a way for us to talk about what we are experiencing now – sharing the good and the bad, our hopes and our anguish, our dreams, and our prayers. The List has brought a group of disparate individuals from around the globe together... as a family.

From Belgium to America

First, a bit about my biological family. My father Philippe was born in Antwerp, Belgium in 1928. His parents Emmanuel and Rebecca were both born in what is present-day Poland. They were introduced by cousins, and ultimately married in 1924 with a Jewish ceremony in Antwerp, followed by a civil ceremony a month later in England. After the wedding Rebecca, who was living in England at the time and Emmanuel, who at the time resided in Germany to avoid the Polish draft, settled in Belgium. Dad didn't speak about any of his life experiences before he arrived in the United States – no family stories, no school stories, no stories about friends or his neighborhood – while I was growing up, he shared no memories with me or my brother at all. Looking back, it seemed that he just wanted to fit in and fly below the radar, so to speak.

My mother Charlotte (named Charnia at birth) was one of three children born in the United States to immigrant parents who were seemingly untouched by the Shoah. She didn't know much about her parents' lives either. I know that her father Morris arrived here with his parents and siblings from Poland in 1912; similarly, her mother Rose arrived with her large family in 1920 from White Russia. Morris entered the Army the day the First World War ended, and only served for four months. Afterwards he was a restaurant owner for a time, and then was a waiter. We don't know if it was an arranged wedding, but they married in 1925.

I lived in a rather strict household and I wasn't about to pester Dad, nor did I know at the time how important his story would become to me in future years. The only time he shared any information with me was for a sixth-grade English assignment, when I had to write a composition about a personal hero. It was only after some prodding from my mom that he briefly recounted a story about how he and his family were imprisoned in and escaped from a Belgian work camp. But after sharing that one story he became silent again. And to respect his wishes or for some other reason still unknown to me, no other surviving family members would share information either. Although I saw them regularly when growing up, neither his sister, his mother; his uncles nor his grandfather would provide any family information. Dad died before I turned 17, two months before my brother's Bar Mitzvah. I left Long Island the day after the Bar Mitzvah to fly to Doxato. By the time I left Greece I had experienced some veiled antisemitism, and a number of disturbing Shoah stories had been related to me. As a result, my father's story piqued my renewed interest, and my quest for more information began.

I now know that the story he told me, although based in fact, was quite fictional. Did he actually not remember, or was he suppressing certain memories? Was he shielding me from the horror, or did he perhaps want to impress me? I will never know. But at the time I was told a very brief, only partially factual story. As it was told to me, the family was living in Belgium when the Nazis arrived and sent them to a Belgian work camp. They managed to procure false papers that indicated they were Catholics who were related to the famous Dutch painter Peter Paul Rubens. My uncle managed to obtain their release, and they left for America. In my eyes, the fact that my father survived this ordeal made him a hero.

In truth, I later found out that in 1942 my father, his sister, and their parents moved from Antwerp to a gentile neighborhood in Brussels, Belgium. What made them so fearful that they adopted false names, obtained false passports and papers, and lived as Catholics while planning to escape and meet other family in England? The Germans had arrived. Emmanuel was an artist who had painted murals in a number of churches, and apparently used the knowledge he gained over the years to teach his family the catechism and some prayers, as well as information about the saints. My father became Philippe Gérard Rubens, shown as a 16-year-old on his forged passport so he would be old enough to have official-looking documents if stopped by the Germans. Along with their new identities, the family also created a false extended-family, and stopped speaking Yiddish.

This was not their first attempt to escape; in 1940 the family spent one month in France but returned to Antwerp when they were unable to escape to England. In 1942 the family split up, with plans to ultimately meet up over the Swiss border. My grandmother and aunt were briefly arrested by a German border patrol, but after a few days and a harrowing period of imprisonment they were released. My grandfather Emmanuel was also arrested and spent several days in prison in Lyon, in unoccupied France. After several days he was released, saved because of his false passport and knowledge of the saints. He then met up with my father Philippe, and they travelled together first to the Belgian consulate and then to Chateauneuf-les-Bains, which at the time was a work camp and training ground for Belgian soldiers in France. After a traumatic train ride the women were reunited with my father and grandfather at the camp, where my father was Bar Mitzvah. Eventually they were ordered to move to Riom, where they lived semi-normal but somewhat primitive lives, albeit as Christians, until France was liberated in August 1944. They moved to Paris and remained in France until 1946, when they obtained papers and left for America. Once again, they were separated for the journey, arriving at different ports on separate ships at different times.

I look at the pictures I have that were taken before the war, and all I see is a normal family enjoying life while performing day-to-day activities – school pictures, pictures of family members smiling while walking down the street, pictures of them enjoying time on the beach. Yet the war changed everything. I also have a picture of my father wearing the yellow star. Although it is undated, it was probably taken before 1942, and his demeanor couldn't be more different. By the time the war was over, 13 relatives who had relocated and were living in Antwerp were gassed in Auschwitz, and most family members remaining in Poland were killed as well. Eleven were imprisoned in the Warsaw Ghetto; most died there or in Treblinka. Yet my father and his immediate family had the foresight to remove all Jewish identification, take up false identities, and flee during the height of the war. Despite many obstacles, they found a way out. In my mind they are all heroes.

But the story doesn't end there. Although my father was not naturalized until 1952, in 1951 he enlisted in the Army. After serving a year at Fort Dix he married my mother, and was ultimately sent to Hoerst, Germany. What was he thinking? After fleeing persecution and losing much of his family, he returned to Europe to help with post-liberation activities. Yes, the war had ended six years earlier, but weren't the memories still too raw, still too painful?

My father was fluent in English, French, German, Yiddish, and Flemish, so he applied to be an interpreter for the army. Despite his language proficiency, his application was denied because he was an immigrant from Belgium, and the government felt that he could not be trusted. This was unacceptable to my parents, so they fought the ruling, and months later somehow managed to get the decision overturned. Several months after my father's departure for Germany, my mother obtained a 30-day visa, with plans to join him there. She took the civil service exam to get a government job, and because of her typing skills she became the secretary of one of my father's commanding officers, enabling her to stay in Germany despite her visa status. And so, they lived and worked together in Germany, and volunteered every weekend for the Jewish Welfare Board at the displaced persons' camp at Föhrenwald. Dad became a language instructor, and they spent a year working together to locate and reunite children with family members. Föhrenwald was a community of sorts, and they were a part of it. To this day my mom recounts the story of red-haired, freckle-faced young sisters who they wanted to adopt and bring home with them. Although their mother had given them up for adoption because she had tuberculosis, the girls were not allowed to enter this country.

Upon returning from Germany, Philippe and Charlotte moved in with her parents in the Bronx until they ultimately found their own apartment. But Carle Place beckoned.

Life Before The List

I grew up in Carle Place, a one-square mile unincorporated village on Long Island with few Jewish families and only one black family. Carle Place was developed by William Levitt as the first prototype low-cost community for returning veterans and their families. I have no memory of antisemitism or bigotry while growing up. There weren't many Jews in this community of little more than 7,000 people, but we seemed to be treated ok. We were and still are a tight-knit community, although apart from High School reunions most contacts are online now. Even back in the sixties and seventies, when we asked the Board of Education to adapt the school calendar and schedule the High Holidays as non-school days, they agreed. They even included a menorah in the High School main lobby's holiday display, next to the Christmas tree.

Family played an important part in my life; we were a close-knit family. Aunt Lily (my father's sister) and her family lived around the corner from us; we moved to Carle Place to be near them. I never knew my dad's father – my grandfather, who died before I was born – but every week we would visit the other grandparents in different parts of the Bronx. When my father's mother moved to Miami Beach, we drove down on an annual trek to visit her. And we would spend every Thanksgiving with members of our extended "British" family on Long Island, hosted by Uncle Mark, the uncle who helped sponsor my father's coming to the States. Uncle Mark owned a ladies' clothing design and manufacturing company, and both my father and Aunt Lily's husband worked there for many years, alongside other Shoah survivors. My parents also participated in a "cousin's club" with relatives from my mother's side of the family, but children were excluded from those gatherings.

I grew up in a Conservative Jewish household. I never dated in high school and I was not permitted to attend my senior prom since I was only allowed to date Jewish boys. There weren't any Jewish boys my age at the school and crossing school boundaries for prom was unheard of back then. But my life was infused with both Judaism and Jewish activism. We kept kosher at home and I regularly attended shul. I often led Junior Congregation services, and as a teenager I sang in the adult choir. I attended Hebrew School and Hebrew High School and was Bat Mitzvah. I was an active member of United Synagogue Youth, serving on numerous regional and national boards. I participated in numerous rallies supporting Soviet Jewry, including several at the Soviet Embassy on Long Island. Back in the day I was even appointed as a youth member to a United Synagogue committee charged with developing a responsa to the question of female involvement in all aspects of synagogue leadership. But back then, at least in my extended community, I can't recall any mention or recognition of the Shoah. We didn't learn about it in public school, and didn't hear about it in Hebrew school, where virtually all the teachers were Israelis who taught either ancient Jewish history or more recent Israel history.

Dad died before I turned 17. He had rheumatic fever as a child which weakened his heart, and he died when he was only 43 years old. His death traumatized me; back then there was no emergency number to call for help. I still remember running down the street to the fire chief's house for assistance until the ambulance arrived. Would he have lived if he had gotten to the hospital sooner? I'll never know, but I always felt guilty, which caused me to question my relationship with such a seemingly cruel G-d. Coupled with what I had just learned in Greece, I really was unsure where my religious life would take me.

When I left Long Island for college, I was looking for a vibrant Jewish community, thinking that might help me in my personal struggle. I found it in Philadelphia. As a result, I now have a joint degree in History and Jewish studies and a Master's Degree in Education from the University of Pennsylvania. Besides non-Jewish activities I was heavily involved at Penn Hillel, and served as co-President of ATID, a region-wide college youth group sponsored by United Synagogue. I taught Hebrew school for several congregations. It was while I was teaching Hebrew School in college that I began to think of myself as a 2g. It started with researching different aspects of the Shoah to bring it closer to the students; it ended with me exploring my own background.

I met my husband Barry through ATID and married him after graduation. We lived in Philadelphia for 18 years, during which time I taught at a Jewish day school and was a Public School substitute teacher until landing a government job, and I also served as a Hebrew School teacher and principal. When we moved to Maryland, I continued teaching in Hebrew schools, and I was a founding member of our new synagogue and co-founder and co-Director of our award-winning Talmud Torah.

Barry doesn't really understand how important family, family history, and Judaism are to me. His back story is very different; both his parents were born in America, and he was falsely told that all his grandparents were as well.

In truth, only the grandmother he knew was born here. Although he attended Hebrew School and his family belonged to a Conservative synagogue, it was not an innate part of his development. And there has been so much family drama that he has little contact with any remaining relatives apart from his sister, her family, and a few cousins. So, there really is no natural family connection. Thus far, our son Phil seems equally disinterested in his heritage, so his deeper familial connection is missing right now as well. I have a hard time understanding why Phil apparently has little regard for his religion. He attended a Jewish day school as an elementary student, attended synagogue, participated in USY, and went to a Jewish overnight camp. We never pushed him. Yet now, as an adult, he seems to have rejected most things Jewish. I understand that in the current environment many millennials are religiously unaffiliated, but I hope he will recognize the value of religion and be drawn back, perhaps once he has children. Neither Barry nor Phil understands how much this pains me. I can't understand why they have such indifference toward family and religion. For me it's quite the opposite. For example, when I was contacted on Ancestry.com about a potential family overlap with a previously unknown family line, I couldn't wait to contact that person for more information, to determine a possible family relationship.

Alex Haley once said, "In every conceivable manner, the family is a link to our past, and a bridge to our future." That was my journey. My family was indeed both a link to my past and a bridge to my future. But I was still searching for fulfillment. That search led me to The List.

My Connection with The List

In May 2008 Phil graduated from high school in Maryland, and he immediately began preparations for his first year of college in Massachusetts.

He had been living home with us for 18 years although he had taken some short trips away from home. For several summers he went to overnight camp. He travelled to Israel twice – once on a Birthright trip, and once as a member of a JCC inaugural high school Maccabi basketball contingent from across the United States that traveled and played games throughout Israel. He also spent two weeks in the Midwest as a Student Ambassador under the People-to-People program. But after those short stints he always returned home. As parents of a serious athlete, Barry and I spent years travelling together to his sporting events, including a trip to San Antonio to watch him excel in the Maccabi games. Phil was named after my father Philippe – now, like my father, he wouldn't be around to talk to regularly. I knew that as soon as he became immersed in his college classes and his new friends and activities, his daily contact with home would cease. And I had no way of knowing if he would return home after graduation. I could already feel a void in my life.

Whether it was coincidence or fate, that was the moment when my cousin invited me to join the 2g List. Hannah, Aunt Lily's daughter, was already a member. She explained that she had joined a children of survivors group several years earlier, and thought I might be interested in participating as well. After thinking about it, I decided to see what the group was all about. I introduced myself briefly via email, and everyone was incredibly welcoming to me. I was initially known to the members on The List as the self-proclaimed "lurker." An introvert by nature, I felt uncomfortable, thinking I didn't really belong. The group had already been together for a number of years, and everyone already seemed to know each other fairly well. When my cousin brought me in, I was apprehensive – I didn't know what to expect, and I didn't even know if I would be accepted as a member.

Except for a few times when the number of messages and information became overwhelming, I read all the messages with great interest. But I felt out of place, and rarely shared information or commented on what I read. At the time I was not comfortable discussing my personal stories with people I had never met, perhaps because it was Hannah who brought the stories to light for me. Dad never shared his experiences – maybe that's why Aunt Lily decided to start sharing her stories with the extended family, so that the family legacy would not be lost forever. It was Hannah who ultimately spent hours speaking with her mother, and it was Hannah who published several manuscripts memorializing those stories. So, in my heart, I considered those stories to more appropriately be Hannah's to share.

Surprisingly to me, at some point Hannah dropped off The List. I don't really know why and I'm not sure she does either. I'm also unsure when it happened. But I know that the pandemic changed my overall perception of family. I now believe there are two types of families – those who are related by birth or family connection – like Hannah and I were – and those who choose to be together, held together by a different type of bond. No longer having the ability to spend time with related family members outside of my home, and eager for contact, zoom gatherings provided me the opportunity to "meet" List members that at the time I only knew superficially and via email. In some respects, members on The List have now become part of my extended family. Yes, we are from different backgrounds and from different countries. We have a variety of interests, diverse life experiences, and different points of view on many topics. By trade we are featured speakers, writers, professors, teachers, historians, psychologists, public servants, and more…a disparate group of individuals, all with different stories to tell, and all joined together through The List.

Though we have many differences, we are held together by an innate understanding of each other's unique backgrounds as children of survivors.

From my perspective, The List has gone through some interesting transitions. There were periods with numerous ongoing discussions of interest to the members. Members voiced concern about serious family illnesses among the members, and talked and supported each other around work problems and difficulties they were having with their grown children. Yet, at other times, The List seemed to be phasing out, with it being quiet for weeks at a time, and individuals only responding to directed questions.

Although members are for the most part respectful toward others' beliefs and opinions, that was not always the case. Some topics brought out both the best and the worst among List participants. What was the biggest disagreement I remember? It occurred soon after I joined The List, and it quickly got ugly. It revolved around intermarriage and started with a shared article equating Jewish marriage with survival of the Jewish people. The posting affected List members differently, but it led to a great deal of vitriol, name-calling, hurtful language, and hard feelings. I believe it also led to several long-time members leaving because they felt that they and their views were disrespected. Some members shared negative and at times seemingly xenophobic views which were certainly hurtful to our intermarried members. It was hard for me to understand why anyone would call intermarried individuals *goyim* who were less than Jewish, particularly since we were all 2g'ers whose families went through similar circumstances. But did I speak out? No, like many members I remained quiet. But I told myself it was because I was new to The List and didn't want to be seen as interfering. Should I have spoken out? Yes, most certainly.

Through the years The List has also served as a support system, as well as a research aide. In the past, members have provided historic information about the Shoah, asked and answered research questions, and shared links to books and oral histories. This was particularly helpful to me when I was looking for information on Belgium, and one of the former List members was able to provide some needed information and context.

More recently, with Hamas sending rockets into Israel, I found myself checking messages regularly for updates on The List members and their families who live there, wanting to ensure they were all safe. I felt relieved when the cease-fire was announced, for the entire country but more specifically for my new extended family. When one person hurts, we all hurt.

Through email we've celebrated family simchas together and supported each other through tragedies. We've shared stories, articles, books and videos, as well as our hopes and dreams through different perspectives. We've prayed for each other and with each other. We may not be related, but we have chosen to be together as family, joined together by our stories, our hopes, and dreams.

Epilogue – From Generation to Generation

Doctor Who, a time traveler and favorite science fiction character, has a background shrouded in mystery. The Doctor travels in a TARDIS, a time machine that appears to be bigger on the inside than it is on the outside. That is also my box, my story through time. At the onset my story was concealed in a mysterious wrapped box, and I had no idea what secrets were contained in it and what might be uncovered when the box was opened. As I completed more research, more layers of the box were unwrapped, but the box kept growing larger. And as the box has grown, so has my story. Will I ever know the entire story? Probably not, but that won't stop me from trying to unpeel more layers. Do I wish some parts of my life had gone differently? Did I fail to unearth some parts of my heritage? Without a doubt – but other pieces have filled some of the void.

Do I regret not becoming involved in The List earlier? Most certainly, because I miss the deep connection that others on The List have. Although I have been a member since 2008, to date I have not met any members of The List in person, yet I believe most others have. I was envious when some members of The List met up in Israel, as well as when another group gathered in New York City. I sense a strong camaraderie amongst members on The List, something I am missing. I am hopeful that in the future I will be able to get together with some members here in the Northeast. But for me, emails and zoom will have to suffice until then.

Why did I stay if I was so uncomfortable during some of the early back-and-forth? Simple – to me this community was a microcosm of the world at large. Regardless of their background and life stories, people have differing opinions on many topics. Whether or not those beliefs match your own, it is incumbent on us to at least listen, and to debate respectfully.

Why am I doing this, and why do I care so much about family? I do this for my brother, who appears to be growing more interested in family history as he gets older. I do it for my son and nieces and nephews – who up until now only seemed to care when they were searching for information for school assignments. They are 3gs who grew up with little overt anti-Semitism, who will need to decide whether to make the Shoah part of their identities. They alone will decide how Jewish they want to be, and what part their family's Jewish history will play in their lives. As they grow older and have families of their own, I am hopeful they will choose to become interested in what made them who they are. I pray that they will take pride in their history and Jewish identity, and in the future will share that heritage with their children. Only time will tell.

Writing this has become a labor of love for me. At first, I wasn't convinced I should participate, or that I had anything to say that would be of interest to anyone other than perhaps my immediate family. I contemplated for several weeks whether to try, but I ultimately decided to add my narrative. And surprising to me, the more I wrote, the more I wanted to express myself and share my story. Participating in this has afforded me the opportunity to delve deeper into my family and heritage, and to share what I have learned.

Writing this has also given me more confidence in myself, which has in turn empowered me, even as an introvert, to speak out when I see or hear about antisemitic, racial, or homophobic incidents. I am much more sensitive when I hear inappropriate remarks or see someone being bullied or discriminated against. I have been a federal employee for over forty years, but the last five years have been the most disheartening of my career. Some of the new political appointees' beliefs were, in my opinion, not grounded in fact, and were the antithesis of the freedoms my family fought so hard for. Adding to that, since the Hamas rocket attacks there has been a large increase in antisemitic and anti-Israel sentiment in the news, in politics, and throughout the world. This has made me much more perceptive to racism, antisemitism and their effect on individuals and the community at large.

And so, I also do this for me. I am in my mid-60s now, and it is important to me that these stories get passed down. My parents and grandparents would have been proud to see the strong woman I have become. I have the strength of my father, who suffered through unspeakable things while surviving the Shoah. And I have the strength of my mother, who left the comfort of her Bronx home and traveled alone to Germany to join my father. My focus continues to be on family, friends, and community; my strength runs deep in all three. Doctor Who travels with a series of companions. My companions are my extended family – my memories and my community. *L'dor va'dor* – from generation to generation.

Dr. Betty Unger Needleman
My 2G Life and My Virtual Community

Introduction

Growing up in Brooklyn, New York, one would think might be a great and perhaps exciting place for a Jewish girl to live. My family was comprised of my parents and my brother, who is five years older than me. My parents owned a family business, a small luncheonette, and they worked extremely long, hard hours. Both were Holocaust survivors from the same small *shtetl* in Poland. My brother attended yeshiva, which I think was an easier place to blend in. After all, many of the other students enrolled in his schools were also children of survivors. As for me, a cousin convinced my mother that public school would be a better environment for me. My mother then persuaded my father to give the local public school a try. After all, why would a little girl need to attend yeshiva? So, in my entire public high school, I can only recall one other girl whose father was also a survivor, and another girl whose grandparents came from the same small town as my parents. The neighborhood was comprised of mostly Italian as well as some Jewish families. The religious neighborhood children obviously attended yeshiva, as did my brother. Most of the other Jewish families in the neighborhood were not affected directly by the Shoah. They did not have accents, like my parents did. They were more Americanized than our family, or so it appeared to me.

My Parents' Origin in their Shtetl Town in Poland

My parents both came from the same small town in Poland that they referred to as Dombrova. Many years later I learned that there are three towns in Poland that go by the name Dombrova! Their town is more formally named Dombrova Tarnowski, or Dabrowa Tarnowksa because it is situated approximately 10 miles from a larger town named Tarnow or Tarnov. My parents simply referred to it as Dombrova. The Jewish community in Dombrova was tight-knit and had a working relationship with the larger non-Jewish members of the community. I believe my parents had a love/hate relationship with the town because antisemitism was always present in their day to day lives.

My mother grew up in a very large family of seven children, and she was the second oldest child. There were six daughters, and the "baby" was a son. He was only seven years old when taken to concentration camp, and my mother thought about him for the remainder of her life, hoping he did not suffer. Their home was very religious, and my maternal grandfather was very well respected. As my mother always said, he was a very scholarly man, and people often turned to him for advice. Still, people complained to him when they saw his daughters ride around town on bicycles, and he was modern enough to tell them to mind their own business when it came to raising his children. He often invited yeshiva boys to their home for a nice Shabbat meal, some meaningful conversation, and probably to introduce his oldest daughters but I am not certain. My maternal grandmother was very busy running the household, cooking, and feeding her large family. Oftentimes my mother and her older sister were delegated to caring for the younger children in the family; that was just expected of them. The family business was selling eggs, maybe even poultry, but I am again not certain. My mother grew up surrounded by a lot of love, near all of her grandparents, aunts, uncles, and many cousins. This is in contrast with my brother and me, who never knew our grandparents. Our cousins were not close in age, but rather, their children were similar in age to us.

My father, on the other hand, was the baby of the family. I believe that he was the sixth child. His mother passed away when he was only two years old, so an aunt who never had children stepped up and took on the responsibility of helping to raise him. There was a wide age spread among the children, and the two oldest brothers moved to the United States when he was very young. In fact, according to my father, they recalled the family dog better than they remembered him. My father did not speak much about his childhood, but I believe it was a happy one. His father passed away prior to WWII and both of his parents were buried in the town's Jewish cemetery. It is still in existence but poorly kept and overgrown. Many of the gravestones were taken by the Nazis during the war years and used for other purposes. Therefore, many of the graves remain unmarked.

Prior to the war my father was a single adult man who was close to his three siblings and their children, all of whom were still living nearby to him. My father always said that he was in the business of "straw and hay". To be honest, I never knew whether there was a difference between them, and I don't recall asking. I do know that he had a good relationship within the Jewish and non-Jewish community. He was a kind and generous man, a people pleaser, who always tried to do the right thing. After my father passed away, I learned from my mother that he traveled up to Warsaw to help the underground fight against the Nazis. He returned home after he was out of ammunition. He never spoke about this to my brother or me.

My mother was about only 15 or 16 years old when things escalated; the Jewish people in her town were rounded up, boarded onto trains, and taken to concentration camp. I learned many years later that it was probably Belzec, an extermination camp. My mother had a strong hunch that there would be a very bad ending, which was matched by her strong desire to live. As she told it, the train she was on slowed down as it went uphill, and she grabbed her opportunity to squeeze through an opening and jump from the train. She tried convincing one of her sisters to jump with her, but that sister refused. My mother had no concrete plan in mind, nowhere to run and hide, as she heard guns fire at others who managed to also jump from the moving train. By a small miracle she was not hit by any bullets, and from then on, she was on her own.

Despite her young age, my mother was very brave, street smart, and fast thinking. These attributes kept her alive for the duration of the war years. She took on the name of a Polish girl, a maid who did not want to leave her family and work family. My mother was not given any formal paperwork to prove her identity, but still managed to fool everyone. She reported to the work camp in place of the maid and was sent to work on railroad tracks in Germany. Growing up in a religious home, she knew very little about other religions but had to pretend to be Christian. She kept a low profile, remained quiet and kept to herself. When others were suspicious, she started going to church. She was always afraid that she might say something that would give her Jewish identity away, like "oy" or "momma". In bed at night, she practiced making the sign of the cross under the covers, so she would do it correctly. When asked why she did not receive mail or care packages like the other girls, she made up stories about her parents being too poor. At confession she didn't know what to do, so she told the priest she was Jewish. Fortunately, he kept her secret.

Towards the end of the war, my mother was in the wrong place at the wrong time. There were sabotage attacks on the railroad tracks. She was found unconscious with many injuries, including a broken jaw, arm, and leg. She woke up in a hospital, with no clear recollection of what had happened. These injuries caused her physical difficulties for the rest of her life, yet she took it in stride, coped, and never really complained, because she was grateful to be alive. As she grew older, the disabilities from her injuries grew worse. By the end of the war my mother was certain she was the only Jew left on Earth.

My father had a good relationship with a farmer in the town and managed to convince him to hide him in his barn. In fact, he hid a group of Jews in the barn. I believe that they all gave him money and their properties as payment for hiding them. Still, they were never surrendered for a reward from the Nazis, as other farmers did. The farmer's wife was not so thrilled about this collection of Jews in the barn, mainly because she was concerned about the safety of her own children. The farmer had some type of special radio or perhaps CB, which was strictly prohibited, and whenever they received news that the Nazis were nearby, sent the Jews out to fend for themselves. No matter if it was bitterly cold or even if there was snow on the ground, out they went. I do understand the farmer and his wife's thinking and actions as the Nazis would have killed everyone, including their family. Still, as a result of hiding in an unheated barn throughout the war years, my father contracted TB and probably pneumonia several times. He had compromised lungs for the remainder of his life.

Immediately after the war my father, who was not a tall man, had difficulty standing up straight and adjusting to the light after crouching in the darkness of the barn during the war years. Ultimately, many years after the war, my father died of emphysema from all his lung infections, even though he never smoked. At any rate, he was forever grateful to the farmer, and sent him holiday cards with money and more for the remainder of his life. I recall one year a daughter was getting married, and my parents went shopping to send fabric to Poland for her gown. My parents even wrote a letter on their behalf after the war, as people in the community were angry with his actions and his accrued wealth from the hidden Jews and wanted to send him to jail.

The Post-war Years

After the war, the few remaining survivors returned to Dombrova hoping against all hope to be reunited with loved ones. My mother hitched a ride home on top of a wagon filled with coal. She described herself as covered in black from the coal, with her hair in pigtails. Upon her arrival she soon learned that she was the sole survivor of her immediate family and perhaps only three cousins in her large extended family survived. Her parents, siblings, grandparents, aunts, uncles, and all other cousins were all killed in the Shoah. To be honest, I don't even know how many extended family members perished, as each family had numerous children. By the conclusion of the war my mother was all of 20 or 21 years old, homeless, had no money, and was alone. My father was able to take back a property, and other returning survivors who had nowhere to go stayed with him. And that is how, despite their age difference, my parents came together.

They stayed in Dombrova for a while, but still felt the antisemitism in and around. They visited the graves of my paternal grandparents in the night, knowing full well they would never return. (Little did they know that one day, many years later, I would go to Dombrova.) They lived in Paris for about a year. Cuba was willing to let Jews in after the war, and they secured the paperwork to go there. But my father really wanted to be reunited with his older brothers who helped secure paperwork for them, and ultimately my parents came to the United States. Although my parents thought about starting a family, my mother felt very strongly about waiting until they left Europe.

They settled in New York City, near my two uncles, their wives, and families. My father felt very strongly about not taking any handouts upon their arrival in America. Like many Europeans, my parents were multilingual, but they did not know any English. My father set out to go to work immediately, and for a short time, my mother attended night school to learn English. With time and practice, both improved their English skills. They knew it was important to know English to succeed in their new home, America. They took jobs wherever they could find work, in their burning desire to reclaim some normalcy to their lives.

One of my father's earliest jobs was working at Nathan's in Coney Island. I believe he worked alongside the original owner. My mother took on factory work. Eventually, my mother became pregnant with my brother, and she felt very strongly about purchasing a business so that they could stop working for others. She spoke about how difficult it was schlepping a young toddler along to look at businesses, and how my brother, a new walker, once fell and hurt himself at one such business. Despite my father's hesitancy, she pushed him into purchasing a small luncheonette in Brooklyn, and they worked in that small mom and pop store for decades to come. My father was especially proud of how they started with nothing and were able to become independent. Once they felt more established financially, I was born five-and-a-half years after my brother. They felt complete, having a son and a daughter. Both of us were of course named for the grandparents that we never knew.

Brooklyn and Beyond

My mother always told me I was very independent, even as a very young child. My parents were busy working long, hard hours in the store. Eventually they even purchased a rental property in the neighborhood, which was their second business. We were middle class; never rich but certainly not poor. Our parents were always there for my brother and me, out of necessity we were both very resilient. This is probably very common for 2gs (Second Generation) like us. To be honest, overall, this has served us both well. I guess it builds character. School was always important. My brother went to yeshiva through 12th grade, and I continued in public school. I loved participating in school activities. Many of my friends were Jewish. My father was always very watchful of us, as he did not want either of us to date non-Jews. Eventually, my brother and I both went to college and additionally, earned higher degrees. In contrast, neither of our parents had formal educations, but rather both were blessed with common sense, good instincts, and very strong survival skills. They were "street smart." Even during happy times, such as my brother's bar mitzvah, and our weddings, I found that there was sadness and a sense of loss mixed in with the happiness. Although as a child I couldn't put my finger on it, I have come to realize there were always ghosts present in the background.

As previously mentioned, there was a large age difference between my parents. As a result, my father was more old-fashioned and traditional while my mother appeared a bit more contemporary. After high school, at the age of only 17, I couldn't wait to spread my wings and fly away. I yearned for my college experience to be an adventure. Most children of survivors attended a local college and commuted from home. Brooklyn College was the school my very traditional father assumed I would attend. In his mind, girls did not venture far from home, away from the watchful eye of their parents. Furthermore, Brooklyn College was the school my brother attended.

I begged to be allowed to attend a state university that was an eight-hour drive from home. To be honest, I had no idea that the state of New York was so large! I had never before traveled more than a few hours from Brooklyn and did not realize that my school of choice was so far from home. But it offered course work in subjects that I was interested in studying and seemed perfect to me. Mind you, I learned this from a catalogue on my guidance counselor's shelf but had never actually visited campus. This was many years before the start of the internet and google, where students today begin exploring all that universities have to offer. I had done some volunteer work while in high school and decided that I wanted to go into a "helping profession" such as physical or perhaps occupational therapy. From my observation, I believe that many 2gs like me have this desire to go into professions whereby we can help others in one way or another and perhaps "make a difference". The State University of New York at Buffalo offered both courses of study, and I begged my mother to let me go. She trusted me, worked on my father to let me go, and ultimately enabled me to go away to college. And so, the "adventure" began.

Although my original plan was to become a physical or occupational therapist, I changed my mind slightly along the way. I did not stray too far, but instead majored in speech pathology and audiology, which is part of the family of professions within rehabilitation. I met my husband during our last year at SUNY at Buffalo. After graduation, we both took some time off to work in the "real world", see where our relationship would take us, and figure out the next chapter of our lives. Then off I went to Ohio to earn a master's degree in Audiology, which I still practice to this day.

Ultimately, my husband and I got married while he was still in school, and we initially lived in Philadelphia, Pennsylvania. Sadly, my father passed away several years after our wedding. Although we loved living in Philly, we eventually decided to relocate closer to our families. My husband and I wanted to start a family. In stark contrast to me, he had fond memories growing up and having a warm, loving relationship with his grandparents. I had a wish for my future children to have that same loving relationship with my mother and in-laws. We were only about 100 miles away, but realistically knew that we would be the ones going back towards New York rather than anyone traveling to visit us. So, we moved to New Jersey and exactly one year later had our first baby boy. Then, two-and-a-half years later, we welcomed our second baby, another son.

While I continue enjoying the professional work that I do, having children is the most important thing that I feel I have done with my life. Our sons have brought so much joy and meaning to me and make life better. Although my husband and I attended public schools growing up, we enrolled our boys in a conservative day school through 12th grade. They grew up with a strong sense of pride in Judaism and love for Israel, which was very important to us. The boys had a warm and loving relationship with their Bubbe (my mother) and their paternal grandparents. Their Bubbe was often more open to sharing stories about the war with my sons than she had been with my brother and me. I believe that as she got older, she didn't want the story of her life and her family to be gone forever. She had fun playing hide and seek with them when they were small and later sat around the table playing Uno as she (and they) got older.

Our younger son went on a trip with his high school to Poland and then Israel. I cried at the airport dropping him off at Lot, the Polish airline. It was still winter, the sky was a bleak and dreary gray, and very cold. He was really overwhelmed being in Poland, as he was well aware of his Bubbe's stories. His mood lifted entirely when he arrived in Israel. Then, about nine years ago, I found myself on a Lot airplane headed for a "heritage trip" with a local synagogue. I refer to it as my "trip *NOT* vacation". It was an eye opener traveling from Warsaw, down through Lublin, and finally to Krakow. Of course, we stopped at cemeteries, forests, and fields where Jews were murdered, and concentration camps along the route, including Majdanek, Plaszow and of course Auschwitz-Birkenau. The tour leaders knew of my family background, and even met my mother who was still alive at that time. They offered to make a stop in the town of Dombrova because the large synagogue there was recently refurbished from disrepair into a beautiful cultural museum.

Although it was so many years after the war and the Nazis were long gone, my mother begged me not to go anywhere alone. She feared for my safety, all these years after the war. My mother remembered the address of the house she stayed in with my father and other survivors after the war and I was able to locate it. My parents had been married in this house! It felt surreal and was very humbling walking around in the town where my family members walked many years ago. The cemetery where my paternal grandparents were buried is still there, but in great disrepair. It was here that I again felt the presence of ghosts from family members who were lost.

Our sons eventually went to college and are now gainfully employed and working hard. My mother had the joy of attending our oldest son's wedding and was so happy to be a part of the *simcha* (celebration). He and his wife now have two small and amazing children of their own. While our oldest son was named for my father, his daughter is named for my mother.

While my sons were still in high school, I went back to school and earned a clinical doctorate degree virtually (online) in a program specifically designed for people like me who are actively working in the field. For most of my career I have worked at a rehabilitation hospital nearby to my home. Additionally, I am employed as a clinical instructor in a local university audiology clinic, working directly with doctoral students. I guess you can say I am paying it forward to the next generation of audiologists.

The List

I honestly cannot recall how or exactly when I found our 2g listserv many years ago, but I am so glad that I did. I have been a member since at least 2003, likely even before that. I believe that in all probability I stumbled upon it accidentally on the internet. I do recall requesting to become a member and feeling honored to be accepted. I did not know any of the members beforehand. I loved that the members were from all around the globe, and the common thread was that somehow the Holocaust bound us together. It is because of our commonalities that I felt the members "got me", similar to the bond one has with old friends. My life is better and richer since I became a member of this 2g List. While my mother feared at the conclusion of the war that she was the only Jew left on earth, this List has shown me that there are others who may feel or think similarly to me, as we have all been touched in one way or another by our parents' experiences.

I prefer not to mention specific names, but I am sure people will recognize themselves in my writing. Some members had parents who were prisoners in a variety of concentration camps, while my parents managed to escape that hell. They lived in their own unique versions of hell. Some had their numbers tattooed on their arms, while others did not. Some members are religious, while some are more secular. Some List members are older than I am, and naturally in different chapters of their lives, while some are closer in age to me. Some never married, some were divorced, and some are widowed. Some had large families, which sounds really lovely, while others had smaller families like me. Some already had grandchildren while I was still busy raising my sons. Some never had children. I have learned different and valuable lesions from each of the members. Many are retired, while I am still working. I have attended a few group events in people's homes, and it is always lovely putting a face to people's names and emails.

One woman, in particular, travels a great distance because she wants to meet the other members and have a more intimate relationship with them. The meetups in homes feel more like a family gathering. Members are very welcoming, the food is always delicious, and the stories previously told come to life in a very special way. One was in a members' home in the Bronx, and another was in Brooklyn. I initially met one member at the campus Hillel when our children began freshman year at the same university. I recall her daughter address us as "family friends" and I felt that was very sweet. Another time, a member who lives in Canada traveled to New Jersey to give a seminar about her work with Holocaust survivors and other related topics. The location was only 45 minutes from my home, it gave me the opportunity to meet her, and of course, her lecture was interesting. I had the opportunity to meet another List member who was also in attendance, which was a bonus.

I feel sad when members face serious difficulties and loss (such as losing a loved one), go through other personal struggles (such as their illness or that of a family member) or face other personal hardships. Group members have felt comfortable enough reaching out to the group and asking us to offer up prayers in support. This act of love and caring stretches across the globe. Greetings are always conveyed during Jewish holidays such as Rosh Hashanah, Yom Kippur or perhaps Passover. It is like being in a special cousins' club.

I dislike when people within the group have disagreements and hate it when members drop out as a result. It makes me feel very powerless as I don't know how to fix the mess or heal the hurt. We all have our own religious beliefs, political beliefs, maybe even personal agendas in life. People get insulted, or may feel threatened, or misunderstood. Let's face it, there is no right or wrong in many of these issues, and how each of us lives our lives is a personal decision. We live in the grey rather than the black and white, and we are all evolving due to experiences in our daily lives. There is no right or wrong way. When writing and participating in an online forum, messages and thoughts are often misconstrued. Then people need to back pedal, or apologize, or explain. But the pain and hurt has already taken hold. The bickering has always made me uncomfortable and during these times I find that I lurk rather than appear to choose sides or even chime in. At other times my own life is just too busy due to work or family commitments and I lurk rather than participate. The "conversation" is so quick and by the time I can participate, the group is on to the next subject line. Then, when I do have the time, the topic may no longer be relevant. The group has already moved on.

I received the emails individually rather than in digest form, because I felt it would be easier to stay current, receiving them when they are actually written and "sent". Sometimes the group goes silent, and I wonder – where did everyone go? Is everyone ok? But eventually someone posts an email that causes the group to come alive again, and responses begin flooding my in-box. The conversation begins again, renewed and refreshed.

In some ways we are like a family, a large family living across several continents. Several members have passed away. I have now attended a virtual funeral. Although we never met personally, while attending the funeral I learned so much about her. Others have disappeared out of personal choice, or because of a disagreement they have had with other members. Tempers flare. I often think about them and hope they are doing well. Some have left the group for a variety of personal reasons or time constraints of their own and have later returned. Some never re-emerge or return only to disappear yet again.

While I may not express it, I really do enjoy when members return to The List. It is like a family that one simply cannot quit. Our recent virtual meet-ups during the pandemic have been lovely. We have worked through ways to connect on zoom, despite the time differences that separate us. Many members have inspired me along the way. One in particular did not know she was Jewish until much later in life. She could have walked away from the whole Shoah mess, but instead decided to dig deeper to learn more. She continues to dig, despite other hardships in her life. Several others have dedicated their entire careers to exploring, teaching, and writing about the Shoah, or writing about their unique family Shoah stories. Others have become therapists with a focus on the Shoah. I admire them for this.

I have tried to "recruit" some personal 2g friends to The List. My brother is aware of The List, to some degree. He always said he was too busy working to get involved. I know that during his quiet moments he does his own exploring on the internet about Shoah related information. But he doesn't have an interest in becoming a part of The List. One friend is a member of the Facebook groups for 2g and finds that it satisfies her personal needs. Thus far, I have not become involved in Facebook at all, but perhaps after I retire from work I will have more time to explore the groups. I always wonder why more daughters than sons are involved and am glad we do have a few male members as they can give a slightly different perspective. Otherwise, I only have a few personal friends who are also 2g. As previously mentioned, my cousins are not 2g, as their parents immigrated to the United States prior to the outbreak of WWII.

One of the things I recall personally sharing about myself with The List is when I earned my clinical doctorate degree. I felt bad that I was lurking but not actually participating in the conversations being shared. The conversations were always important to me, and I read each and every one of the emails. I felt guilty about lurking, but there are just so many hours in the day. In addition to school, I was working, raising the boys, running them to/from their activities, carpooling, and trying to get meals on the table. During school breaks we visited colleges they were interested in applying to. My husband joked that people in our synagogue were convinced we were getting a divorce because he frequently went to events without me. When asked where I was, he felt people did not believe when he told them I was home doing my school assignments. The look on their faces said it all – oh sure, she's home doing her schoolwork! It felt good to get back to my life after those two long years. It felt good to get back to The List as well.

I shared with the group about my heritage trip to Poland. It impacted upon me in so many ways that words cannot describe. It was a painful and eye-opening experience for me. Looking back, I am glad I went there while my mother was still alive. I wish I had more time to spend in my parent's shtetl town, perhaps explore town records about my family. I also regret that I couldn't travel to what remains of the Belzec Concentration Camp, where my mother's family most likely perished. My trip inspired another List member to also go on a similar trip to Poland.

Another very important event, the most important of all, was sharing when my mother passed away. I thought and hoped she would live forever and was crushed when she was gone. After all, in many ways my mother was a superhero. People talk about how one day there will be no survivors left to tell their story, and that is something I did not want to face. My mother was very sick for about five weeks, going from the hospital to "rehab". It was so exhausting running and crying, crying, and running. And praying. I just didn't know what to do first, but most of all, my brother and I desperately wanted her to recover. I was not ready to let go, and honestly, I don't think I ever would be. I knew the group would understand and be there for me, and the words from others who had been through this before were very comforting.

Finally, it has been lovely to share the news of the births of my grandchildren. Our granddaughter is now three years old, and her baby brother just celebrated his first birthday. They are simply such a delight! As an adult I have come to realize what a miracle it is that my brother and I were ever born in the first place, after all that our parents went through during their war years. Now there are 10 miracles – my brother and I, our children, and grandchildren. Without my parents' fortitude, and of course luck, none of us would be here today.

Prof. Judith Tydor Baumel-Schwartz
My Life in Lists

Introduction

I love order. My clothes hang neatly in my closet, arranged by category, length, and color. My desk always boasts a precisely folded "to do" list of tasks. Order is security, safely, control over your life. One day, it might even save your life. You don't get it? Just ask a child of Holocaust survivors, like me. They will explain it to you.

I wasn't always like that. Until I was 12 my room was a G-d- awful mess and I never took notes in school, relying on memory. But eventually the "now you are an adult, you are a Bat Mitzvah girl" speech, hit home. As an only child I realized that not only must I take charge of my life, but I might suddenly have to take charge of my parents' lives as well. After all, you never know when you'll have to pick up and run, so your stuff had better be in place, making it easier to grab before you go. It even pays to have a list of what to take ready on your desk. Even better, have a bag packed in your closet with important documents, hard cash, and a change of clothes. "Cash? Never!" exclaimed a 2g ("Second Generation") friend in all seriousness when she heard about my bag. "Much too bulky. Only diamonds, best for trading lives!", she concluded, the voice of her parents' wartime experiences. Yeah, she got it.

Once, my sister, whose neatness puts mine to shame, asked me whether I hang my clothes facing the same direction. "Of course!", I answered "Otherwise how can you put something on fast when they bomb you and the power goes out?". She nodded without raising an eyebrow or missing a beat. Of course she did. After all, she was the one who ran. But wait? Wasn't I an only child? Well, yes and no. I am my mother's only child, but I have a half-sister and half-brother on my father's side, born before the war. THE war, as we 2gs have only one war, all others paling in comparison. Unlike my American-born mother who was my sister's age, my half-siblings had been born in Germany and spent their formative years running from Hitler, first to Belgium, then to France, and ultimately to the United States, while their mother was being shot in Poland, and our father was trying to avoid being shot in Buchenwald and Auschwitz. No wonder I thought that order, structure, and lists might give me some control over an uncontrollable world.

Guess what? They didn't. Neither did becoming a Holocaust historian, possibly hoping to keep the cataclysm from recurring. Nor did starting Israel's first, and short-lived, 2g organization in 1980, which rapidly dissolved when I tired of hearing 25-year-olds gripe about their privileged lives. But close to two decades later, when I came across an online private discussion group for children of survivors from all over the English- speaking world, I was in a different place. I was close to forty, had lost my survivor-father in the interim, and could finally concentrate not only on the first generation, but on the second. I started reading, joined, and was hooked. Another list! But of a different kind. Maybe this one would be my salvation.

Family, History, Life, and Everything In-Between

Being almost three decades younger than my half-brother and half-sister, we never lived together under one roof. After all, they were long married and had their own children before I was born. I grew up knowing that without the Holocaust, my father's first wife (my "stepmother" in our family's parlance) would have lived, my father wouldn't have met my mother, and I wouldn't have been born. So actually, I owe my life to the Nazis, those bad guys from THE war, who could always return. Or as my daughter once said, speaking of the Iranian danger: "Nazis. Farsis. Whatever". Each generation and its boogeymen. Yeah well, she got it too. It just depends on who you are and where you come from.

So where did I come from? I spent most of my formative years growing up in Woodside, Queens, but we were anything but your typical American family. Not your typical American Jewish family either, and come to think of it, not even your typical American Jewish Holocaust survivor family, if there was ever such a thing.

On one side we were a family of storytellers. My maternal ancestors were always into family history, and their stories accompanied me from as far back as I can remember. Growing up I heard numerous family stories that stimulated my imagination. I also learned how to identify an unusual story, and my family was unusual on any scale.

My maternal grandmother was a teenager from a Chassidic family when she immigrated to America from Bukovina in 1911. Seventeen years later, deep into spinsterhood, she met my grandfather, a communist-atheist widower with four teenage sons, and the two fell in love at first sight, marrying almost immediately. She and I shared a special bond as we were both "Second Generation" of sorts, her parents having died of starvation in Transnistria in 1942. But she could only tell me stories about their lives until she left Europe and knew few details about their Holocaust experiences. Those I learned from her siblings who remained in Europe throughout the war, and from my mother who heard them from her uncles and aunts.[1]

My mother's father immigrated to America from Kiev in 1906. He also lost a sister in the war, but never spoke to me about it. In fact, he never spoke to me about his European family at all, nor did he ever mention Russia which he had not been unhappy to leave. I heard about my great-aunt who was murdered in Babi Yar, from my mother, who told me that Aunt Mata hadn't immigrated to America with the rest of the family because she heard that one couldn't keep kosher in the New World. Unlike her communist brothers and sisters, she remained traditional, not that it helped her in the long run as she died, and they lived. Food for thought.

Food was always plentiful in my mother's household, but religion was scarce, being a loaded topic in her family. Before they got married my grandparents had agreed that the house would be kosher, my grandmother would remain traditional, and my grandfather and his four sons would behave as they wished. My mother Shirley, my grandparents' only daughter born in the late 1920s, was brought up with a modicum of Jewish tradition, but followed her father's communist ideology. That is, until she met my father, an Orthodox Holocaust survivor twice her age, a widower with two grown children, and her boss.[2]

My father Chaskel Tydor was born at the beginning of the 20th century in Bochnia, a small Polish town in Western Galicia, to a family of Bobover Chassidim. Like many Jews from that area, during the First World War his family became refugees in Germany. Remaining there after the war's end, they kept many of their Chassidic customs but became part of the Orthodox German-Jewish community. During the early 1930s my father married a girl from his Polish hometown, and the couple had two children. They could have had a wonderful life together as a family, but they didn't, because a year later Hitler came to power.

My father's story is a combination of "could haves" that didn't happen. He and his family could have left Nazi Germany for Palestine, as did a few of his friends, but his wife insisted that she wouldn't leave without her parents who were still in Poland, and those parents refused to consider moving

---

1 Judith Tydor Baumel-Schwartz, *My Name is Frieda Sima: The American-Jewish Women's Immigrant Experience Through the Eyes of a Young Girl from the Bukovina*, Bern: Peter Lang, 2017.
2 Judith Tydor Baumel-Schwartz, *For the Love of Shirley: One Woman's Challenges and Choices in Postwar Jewish America*, Bern: Peter Lang, 2020.

to the Holy Land. Instead, my father applied for visas to England where he hoped to find work as an industrialist. They could have moved to England, but the first round of visas came too early for his wife to agree to use, while the second round came too late to save him from five-and-a-half years of Nazi camps, and his wife from being murdered in Poland.

Founding a survivors' kibbutz in postwar Germany and bringing it to Palestine where he lived until 1951, he could have stayed in the newly founded State of Israel and become a book publisher like his childhood friend who had moved there from Germany in 1935. But my father ended up managing a travel agency in New York to be near my siblings, rescued to America in late 1941. There, his Chassidic contacts tried to marry him off to Holocaust widows from notable Chassidic dynasties who were very interested in the middle-aged Orthodox widower. He could have married one of them, but he didn't. Instead, he concentrated on making a living and trying to reconnect with and marry off his two children, then in their early 20s.[3]

Now comes the really interesting part. At some point when his secretary at the travel agency was about to begin her maternity leave, she highly recommended that he hire her girlfriend Shirley who was between jobs. Warning him not to take Shirley's radical politics seriously, she emphasized her typing skills, dedication, and professional devotion, saying that she would probably be willing to put in long hours of work for very little pay. Shirley came for an interview, Chaskel was desperate for a capable secretary, and she began work the next week.

From that point on, my parents' story surpassed that of my grandparents. My mother indeed typed over 100 words a minute, and within a short time, her personal devotion to my father paralleled her professional devotion to the company. My very Orthodox father was seemingly unaffected by the knowledge that his secular\communist secretary was besotted with him, but that state of events didn't last long either. He certainly hadn't planned to fall in love with a young woman half his age – but he did, bringing her chocolate eclairs to the office every evening in lieu of paying overtime while they worked long into the night on clients' itineraries and balancing the office's books. In between, they eventually managed to get to a kosher coffee shop where my father declared his love for her over *mohnstrudel*. Differing in background, belief and temperament, my parents waited almost five years

---

3 Judith Tydor Baumel-Schwartz, *The Incredible Adventures of Buffalo Bill of Bochnia (68715): The Story of a Galician Jew – Persecution, Liberation, Transformation*, Sussex: Sussex Academic Press, 2009.

to get engaged until both of my father's children were married with children of their own, but in our family, love is love, and it eventually conquers all.

As soon as they married my mother adopted the persona of a typical Orthodox Jewish housewife. Well maybe not typical, nor a housewife, but definitely Orthodox, at least in my father's presence. Eventually, she also adopted the persona of a quasi-survivor, "the wannabe" as I irreverently called her, atoning for the fact that by a twist of fate she had been born in America before the war, and not in Europe like many of her cousins who went through the war. Just to make things even more interesting, for the first two years of their marriage my parents moved to the "wild west" – Deer Lodge, Montana, and Rapid City, South Dakota, where my father managed uranium mines. Eventually they returned to New York for my birth, also returning to the travel business where they first met. Did I mention something about an unusual story?

And Now For Me

All this is background to my story. I came into the world in 1959, an aunt to three nephews and a niece even before I was born. I can't remember when I first learned about the Holocaust because as far back as I could remember it was there. When it came to the Holocaust our family had a division of labor. My father told me the hopeful stories while my mother – the only non-survivor in our nuclear family – passed on the real dirt, like my father's wartime horror stories from which he shielded me.

The Holocaust was a constant presence in my home, a story of devastation, but also one of survival and victory. The message "with G-d's help we triumphed over Hitler" was one I embodied in my very being. Many classmates in my Orthodox Jewish Day School were 2gs, most, like me, named for relatives murdered by the Nazis. To whatever degree, we were all "memorial candles" for those who perished, compensating our parents for what they had lost.

When I was 15, my family moved to Israel as my mother had decided that's where we should go. My father, who had lived in Israel between 1945 and 1951, had no objections. On the contrary, he was thrilled when my mother told him a few years earlier to buy an apartment in the Holy Land. Are Holocaust survivors overprotective of their children? Nah, it was just by chance that my father bought an apartment seven minutes away from Bar-Ilan University to ensure I would never have to dorm. Or drove me to college most mornings, so that he wouldn't have to worry about what could happen to me on a bus. Or was majorly concerned about how I would support myself when I chose to study history but refused to pursue a teaching certificate.

"You need both a trade and a profession", my mother would constantly remind me, "one that you can take with you if you have to run." My high school graduation present was a bilingual secretarial course as "typing and shorthand can save your life". "Just think about the 'Secretaries of Auschwitz'", my mother, the American-born "wannabe" survivor, remarked when I showed her my course completion certificate. Whoever says that intergenerational transmission of trauma magnifies with time knows their stuff. My oldest daughter got that same course from me even earlier, as her bat mitzvah present.

The typing course, of course, paid off, and my bilingual office skills served me well in the job market. Within days of graduating from college I was working as personal assistant for a well-known architect, earning a salary beyond my wildest dreams. The money came in handy as I was already supporting two, having married a fellow student, an *Amerikaner* who was pursuing a graduate degree, despite teenage declarations that I would only marry another 2g. The marriage at 19 came in handy to give my septuagenarian father *yiddishe naches* ("Jewish joy"), and the hope that he would live to see my children grow up. But the job was awful, the marriage wasn't heaven either, and the children weren't even a fleeting possibility in my psyche. What could I do? My husband was away on army reserve duty and my level of despair rose daily.

One night I dreamed that I was standing on the ramp in Auschwitz bathed in fog. A train approached and a group of my relatives who had been killed in the war disembarked. Helplessly I watched them being taken to their death and shouted: "wait for me!", but they continued marching into the darkness. Suddenly my grandmother Esther, my father's mother for whom I was named, turned around and said: "My child, remain here. You have a task. To make sure they won't forget us." And then they all disappeared into the fog.

I awoke in a cold sweat, alone in our sweltering apartment. What now? What should I do so to make sure that "they won't forget us"? Like most of my important decisions, my mind went "click" "click" "click" as the puzzle pieces fell into place. I would quit my job, return to school, specialize in the Holocaust, and then write about it and teach it. But what about my being the family breadwinner? That morning I told my boss about the dream and my decision. He listened attentively, leaned back in his chair, and said: "Return to school, study Holocaust, and one day you will be a famous historian." Smiling, he continued: "And I will proudly tell everyone that you were once my assistant!"

My spirits lifted as I registered for graduate studies in Jewish history at Bar-Ilan University, preparing to write about the Holocaust and eventually teach about it. A year later I also co-founded the first Israeli 2g organization, a short-lived long-named enterprise with the unimaginative title: "Organization of Children of Holocaust Survivors in Israel". Why did I need to establish a 2g organization? Was I beginning to realize, like my American counterparts who were about to found similar groups, that we were a bit strange, or to use a kinder term, "unique"? That as 2g writer and critic Melvin J. Bukiet nails it, "no one who hasn't grown up in such a household can conceive it, while every 2g has something in common"?

Actually, no. I had wanted to start a volunteer group where healthy young 2gs would assist indigent aging survivors and dissolved the initiative when it morphed into group therapy without a therapist. Swearing to explode if I heard one more whining 2g complain about their life ("All your sufferings can't compare to an hour in Auschwitz!") I vowed never to have anything to do with 2g organizations. How fortunate for me that pre-Yom Kippur prayers include expiation of vows.

Instead of concentrating on 2gs I returned to studying 1gs (survivors), which I did conscientiously for the next 15 years. There was also my 80-year-old father's unforgettable statement, "It isn't my life's desire to have a grandchild named after me", catalyzing my oldest daughter's birth 10 months later, even before my dissertation was approved. "I had it all figured out", my mother once said when I asked how she dared marry a man 25 years her senior. "You were born when he was 56, would marry when he was 75, and have children by the time he was 80 so he could enjoy them for the next decade." Thank you mother for planning out my life. How amazing that it worked out exactly that way. Wannabe survivors obviously have power by proxy.

Two years later I had a second child (this time without my father's prodding!), finished my degree, and began teaching Holocaust as an adjunct throughout the country, including at the University of Haifa. But I soon realized I needed an escape hatch and began working on Gender and State of Israel Studies as well as Holocaust studies. At the time, my personal and professional life was in flux. I was my family's major breadwinner in a very complex marriage that was becoming more perplexing by the year. I lacked a strong university mentor who could storm the barricades to get me a tenure-track job, and I was publishing non-stop in the hope of being considered for such a job if it ever became available. I also feared that one of the top people in the Holocaust field in Israel, with whom I had worked in the past, would never let me progress past a certain level. To loosen the professional stranglehold, I had to move into uncharted territory. But it was more than that. Without admitting it to myself, I was slowly experiencing "Holocaust burnout".

Fast forward a decade. I already had a steady job, my husband still did not. I rarely saw my daughters awake as I was moonlighting all over the country to support my family. My beloved father, gone at almost 90, had done a good job of bequeathing me my religious grounding, intellectual education, and 2g legacy. My mother, now the official "survivor" by proxy, was doing an equally good job of bequeathing me "her" Holocaust traumas, including her fears about Israel's future.

It was then that I found The List.

The List and I

For the life of me I can't remember exactly how I stumbled upon "The List", but stumbled it was. Like so many moments that change your life, it happened by accident in late 1998 or early 1999, while combing the net in search of sources for an article. In the process, I must have come across a reference to The List, referred to as a "Second Generation (2nd-Gen) internet discussion group", hosted by Shamash, the Jewish network that was a service of Hebrew College in Boston. Today I know that it was founded in 1995 by Paul Foldes who became the moderator\owner of the Shamash 2nd-gen listserv List, but at the time I was clueless as to its history and composition. All I recall is that it piqued my curiosity enough to note its existence and address at the top of the long yellow legal pad kept next to my computer, just like the one on which I had my list of "what to pack just in case." Nothing like being prepared.

Bogged down with work, it took me a while to go into Shamash and read the group's blurb, but when I did, it suddenly looked pertinent – "To provide a forum and mutual support opportunity for adult children and grandchildren of survivors of the Holocaust. It warmly welcomes those who have interest in the topics relevant to this group of persons from around the world."[4] Hmm. Adult children of survivors. All over the world. Warmly welcomes. Relevant topics to discuss. There I was. Or was I?

---

4 https://remember.org/children1/2g.html, retrieved on June 16, 2021.

Unlike my attitude two decades earlier, this time I was ready to focus on myself. Or at least "readier". I entered the waters cautiously as they did not part before me like the Red Sea, but rather forced me to dive in headfirst while gulping for air. Somewhat painful but ultimately invigorating. Even lifesaving. After lurking and reading for a few days, I began to post, initially cautious when writing about my family or my past. Slowly I got to know a few of the group members, who numbered over 100 at the time, half of whom posted occasionally and 25 % of whom were active posters. I already knew one of them, my former student at the University of Haifa, Ruth Samuel Tenenholtz who now became my friend. Other veteran members who had joined before me or around when I did, whose insightful posts often were reminiscent of my own feelings, also caught my interest: Marty Herskovitz. Paula David. Jeanette Friedman. Marilyn Boehm. Deep awareness. Kindred spirits. Future friends.

Meanwhile, like so many organizations, The List's administration was undergoing changes. Having tired of the bickering and personal attacks (nothing like too many Jews in one framework – the "this is my synagogue, this is yours, and this is the one I would rather be dead than step foot into" syndrome) Paul Foldes turned its management over to Jake Goldstein who would moderate for another few years before he, too, would leave, passing it over in turn to Nathalie Klein, Paula David, and others. At some point, The List would also migrate from Shamash to Smartgroups, then to Yahoo groups, and finally, to Google groups where it exists today in a private and unmoderated form.

That series of turnovers and migrations paralleled several of my own, beginning in late 1999. The first was a migration to economic stability and professional advancement, having finally secured a full-time tenure track position at Bar-Ilan. High time for a 40-year-old 2g who craved security from the day she was born. Too bad that it came with a price: a stressful, superfluous gladiatorial battle with another candidate, orchestrated, no less, by my former thesis advisor, also a 2g, but of a very different ilk. My kind of 2gs are strong, resourceful, and know how to fight to the death. After all, we are children of *survivors*, aren't we? Ultimately, I won the battle, and decided to put the regrettable incident behind me as I began teaching my new and challenging students. Unfortunately, however, the body is often weaker than the mind, as I soon found out.

The second migration was less promising, as I moved from the world of the healthy into that inhabited by those with chronic illness. Throughout the autumn of 1999, the stress under which I had functioned for years finally took its toll on my health beginning with a virus, leading to an unremitting low-grade fever, and then to exhaustion that barely allowed me to get out of bed. Initially diagnosed as Chronic Fatigue Syndrome, it was actually an autoimmune illness that would begin developing years later. How ironic that it hit, just as I got a glimpse of economic security awaiting me around the bend. And how depressing that instead of being able to enjoy not having to run around to eight adjunct teaching positions throughout the country as I had done for years, I had to develop strategies to hide my illness from colleagues and superiors to keep my hard-won position and ultimately be awarded tenure three years later. Did I say children of *survivors?* That's what we are good at, absorbing survival strategies with our mother's milk. Yes, the low-grade fever continued throughout that entire period and no, it did not miraculously disappear the week I got tenure. For my body to begin healing, it took much more than that, including several more migrations, but first, let's get back to my burgeoning relationship with "The List".

For the first year after getting sick I was too exhausted to do much more than lie in bed, dragging myself out to teach three times a week and drugging myself with Tylenol to reduce my fever during the hours I had to be in class. But by the end of that school year, knowing that I must "publish or perish" in the academic world, I began another migration, this time to my desk. There I would sit in front of my computer, hunched over in exhaustion, while trying to churn out articles that would secure my future at the university. When in need of a breather, I would first turn to health-related internet forums where everyone wallowed in health issues and that mostly depressed me, and then to "The List" where everyone wallowed in Holocaust issues, which I now found emotionally invigorating. How could that be? I guess everything is relative.

Speaking of relatives, that was another migration. Acutely aware of how tenuous life and health were, I began asking myself what I – not my parents, children, friends, or community – wanted out of the rest of my life. Rethinking some of my relationships, I realized it was time to migrate out of my marriage, where friendship and shared values had never really been enough to create a solid and fulfilling husband-wife bond. My husband and I amicably divorced, remaining good friends until today. Two years later I remarried another divorced academic, my former Dean at Bar-Ilan (another *Amerikaner*...). While I had shared much of my academic tribulations and 2g-related considerations with The List, I deliberately kept my marital deliberations private until after the divorce, as they involved my soon-to-be-exspouse and not just myself. Long ago a friend had taught me that "everyone has the right to 'sell' their own intimacy, but they have no right to 'sell' that of another". As this was not just my story, it could only become a List story once it was over and done with.

Cyber-discussions

So what did I discuss on The List? Everything else under the sun...but in stages. First and foremost, 2g issues. Fears and anxieties, hopes and desires, fantasies and nightmares, which in the early days of The List, we discussed nonstop. What are we most afraid of? (Believe me, you don't want to know...). When did our nightmares begin? (Probably, before we were born). Why are so many of our anxieties related to the Holocaust? (Are you serious?!). Having rarely given voice to these issues, I discovered that when taken out of their deep, dark closet to be examined by List members in the blue light of cyber-world (my first computer screen was actually green), they were suddenly less frightening. "A sorrow shared is a sorrow halved", with List interaction showing it equally true for anxieties, hopes, and dreams, whether we lived in Tuscon, Toronto, Tottenham, or Tel-Aviv. G-d bless The List.

Another popular topic was our parents. During The List's early years, many of us still had parents who were very much part of our lives, sometimes complicating those lives to a degree where their descriptions would have been totally alien to your average non-2g (and certainly non-Jewish) adult. Our discussions showed that our survivor parents (and their non-survivor spouses) may have come in all shapes and sizes, yet so many of their issues (or our issues with them) were connected to you know who, that guy with the little mustache who tried to annihilate us all. Guilt, guilt, guilt makes the Jewish world go round, and the 2g world was no exception. We felt guilty that we didn't spend enough time with our parents, we felt guilty that we didn't have enough patience for them when we did, and we made great efforts to justify not feeling guilty when we griped about our own, often mundane problems, in comparison to those that our parents had when they were our age and younger.

Unlike us, however, our parents could remember a world before the Holocaust, while we were stuck in WWII-land right from the beginning. A good shrink could have made quite a living off us, but we were busy enough shrinking ourselves on The List. "Memorial candles"? As a group we probably composed a bloody candle factory, with so many of us burning ourselves from both ends, as we often noted.

Then there was religion, a "hot potato" on List discussions, if there ever was one. How do we feel about our Jewish heritage and connection to Judaism and Jewish practice\praxis? As 2gs we came in all shapes and sizes. Some of us, like me, were Orthodox, one or two tended to ultra-Orthodoxy, some were Conservative, Liberal, and Reform, while others were unaffiliated. Then there were those who were not Jewish by *Halacha* (Orthodox Jewish law), but were 2gs because of a survivor parent, usually their father. I was initially surprised by this phenomenon, but later learned how common it was, particularly in Eastern Europe. "The first question you should ask a 2g from Poland or Hungary is: 'when did you first learn that you were Jewish?' ", remarked a Polish-Canadian 2g friend when we once spoke about survivor offspring self-identification.

At a certain point, List discussions of mixed marriages in general, and not just children of such marriages, became very personal and volatile, causing a few members to take a step back and examine whether they felt comfortable in present company. Did an accepting attitude towards List members in mixed marriages condone a phenomenon that Orthodox Jews saw as undermining the continuity of the Jewish people? What about mixed marriages where the 2g partner was not *Halachically* Jewish? Suddenly forced to articulate my beliefs on what had been an agonizing topic in my birth family, these discussions catalyzed my reexamining them, this time without my parents' filters and expectations. This exploration opened a door for me to reconsider many of my responses to various situations, as I asked myself whether I had chosen them through intellectual or emotional identification, or just because I was replicating what was expected of me by my parents, family, or community. My response was often surprising, even to me.

Very often, the concept of "community" guides us more ways than we are aware of, and The List was no exception. For any such group to succeed, it must eventually become a community, in this case, a cyber-community. Communities have their positive elements: empathy, closeness, compassion, and mutual assistance. As the years passed, List members began sharing their personal and not only 2g lives. Together we celebrated personal and professional milestones, moves, weddings, births of children, grandchildren, and great-grandchildren. We mourned the losses of jobs, homes, pets, and the tragedies of burying parents, spouses, and children. Eventually, we also mourned List members whose deaths reminded us of our own mortality. Although we still defined ourselves as "children" (of survivors), we were already deep into late middle age and far beyond. Buoyed by our mutual 2g heritage, at times of crisis, we rallied together to act as an enveloping unit, checking in with each other and offering cyber and other assistance when we knew that our members lived in areas plagued by flooding, earthquakes, fires, instability, or war. This was particularly true at times of crisis in the

Middle East, due to the size and closeness of the "Israeli contingent" to which I belonged.

Communities also have their flip side: power struggles, ego issues, personal jealousies, dramas, misunderstandings. While The List had initially made great efforts to avoid issues common to internet forums such as trolling,[5] flaming,[6] and cyberbullying,[7] by the time I became a fully participating "card-carrying" List-member, our online 2g community was already suffering from some of the ills that plague traditional communities.

As 2gs, many of us came to The List with serious emotional baggage, which more than once played a role in our online interactions. The resulting dramas often focused on three or four dominant posters whose online altercations, at various junctures, overwhelmed any attempts at other 2g-related discussions. Throughout the years I watched (and at times participated in) heated discussions that turned personal, after which certain List members would leave (and return, and leave, and return) very vocally. One member was even asked to leave because of repeated personal attacks and anti-social online behavior. Others, unwilling to bare their souls in what they now viewed as a hostile environment, quietly backed out of posting, now to lurk, while a few members backed out of The List entirely, never to return. Depending on the timing and the personalities involved, one or two posters then acted as peacemakers, reaching out offlist to the parties involved. Behind-the-scenes intervention of smoothing ruffled feathers and stroking volatile egos sometimes brought the irate or upset List member back into the fold. At other times, however, nothing would help, and the aggrieved List members would leave for weeks, months or years, sometimes never to return.

In the long run, the positive List interactions far outweighed any other kind. For me, one of the loveliest aspects of our 2g cyber-community was the offline interaction and particularly the face-to-face meet-ups that we had

---

5 People who deliberate provoke others online. See: Yair Amichai-Hamburger and Gideon Vinitzky, "Social Network Use and Personality", *Computers and Human Behavior* 26 (6) (Nov. 2010): 1289–1295.

6 Posting deliberately hostile messages to target specific aspects of a controversial conversation. Yair Amichai-Hamburger, *The Social Net: Understanding Our Online Behavior*, Oxford: Oxford Scholarship Online, May 2013.

7 Characterized by aggression, bashing, and intimidation. Sisi Hu, *Why Cyberbullies Choose Cyberspace: From the Perspective of Uses and Gratifications,* Thesis, Iowa State University, 2016. https://lib.dr.iastate.edu/cgi/viewcontent.cgi?article=6730&context=etd, retrieved on Oct. 25, 2021.

throughout the years in various locations. Many were quite small, when two or three members got together somewhere in the world to meet a traveling poster. Some were planned, but for whatever reason never managed to take place, like my attempts to meet-up with Patrice Flesch when we both visited New York. Other meetings were larger, like the first Israeli get-together at Stam Tish in Tel Aviv in the summer of 2001, when we took over a large upstairs table, and got to know each other as more than names on a List. At a meet-up at Judy Montel's home in Beit Shemesh, soon after the birth of one of her children, we got to see a different part of the country. During more recent get-togethers at the Azrieli mall in Tel Aviv, we met visiting List members from abroad. I often asked myself whether the "Israeli contingent" had a life of its own, due to the common denominators that members living abroad could intellectually understand but never feel as deeply as we Israelis (none of whom were actually born in Israel) did. Yet many of us in Israel also developed close relationships with individual posters abroad. Could it be that our closest relationships were primarily with those List members we had met face-to-face, or with whom we had developed bonds outside The List? And yet, The List, with all it involved, has remained an integral part of our lives, whether we post actively, or lurk, as was seen when everyone was asked to write a few words during the Covid-19 pandemic just to "check in" and tell the group that they were all right.

Epilogue: When a List Is More Than a List

For two-and-a-half decades The List and I have developed in concert. At times it sounded more like a cacophony, but we were nonetheless in accord. Over and over, I felt that my List discussions and involvement with its members continued to parallel shifts and developments in my own life, value-system, and ethical code. Most were connected to my slowly being able separate some of my opinions and values from those of my parents', and particularly those of my mother. High time for it to happen in the sixth decade of my life!

While I didn't make long speeches about my beliefs, my mother, the "wannabe survivor", had been quite vocal about hers, at least to me. Children don't have to be happy. They have to be obedient and do the right thing. Traditions should be kept in order to commemorate all those we lost to Hitler. The right way to be a "good Jew" is how you were brought up. Being a "good Israeli" didn't count, as by then, my mother was already majorly turned off by life in Israel, which she discovered to her dismay, was nothing like Jewish life in South Florida. Toe the line, and I will love you. Otherwise, I don't know your name. Only later would I realize that such declarations were her last ditch attempts to navigate a world in which she was drowning without a lifeline, but then I took her seriously, even when she didn't take herself seriously. Consequently, I adopted many of her values to retain her love and moral support, never really crystallizing my responses to major issues in my life by drawing on my own beliefs, opinions, and personal experiences.

How did I feel about living in Israel? Did I only remain out of inertia or an inability to find a suitable professional position in the Tri-State area? How deeply should I be involved in my children's lives? In what ways should I respond to intermarried friends and family? What is the correct work-life balance? To what degree should elderly parents' needs or wishes take precedence over those of other family members? These were only some of the issues I grappled with during my years on The List.

Headed discussions about patriotism and national feelings of belonging, particularly among our American and Canadian members, led me to ponder the meaning of "homeland", and ultimately helped me clarify my own feelings about living in Israel. Impassioned List debates about the degree to which we can or should be enmeshed in our children's lives, and vice versa, enabled me to better understand the controlling tools that carve out the nature of our dearest relationships. Intense arguments over the scope and impact of intermarriage in the contemporary Jewish world induced me to review my feelings and actions towards the phenomenon in my closest circles. Poignant List conversations about life satisfaction and regret impelled me to reexamine the role that work played in my life, encouraging me to reshape not only my work-life balance, but also rethink the aspects of my profession to which I wanted to devote the remainder of my employment years. Complex dialogues among List members about being the "sandwich generation" made me realize the extent of what I was experiencing, and the impossible choices we were all forced to make. It didn't necessarily make my choices easier, but it did comfort me to know that I wasn't alone in feeling as I did.

Today, the official "List" has shrunk to a third of what it was when I joined in the late 1990s, and the number of active posters rarely exceeds a dozen. Discussions are usually less emotional than they were in the past, as we try not to push each other's buttons. But even if we have lost some of the excitement, we have gained something in return: a sense of fellowship, almost a kinship. Many of those who have remained active are part of each other's lives both on- and off-list. We celebrate together, mourn together, and grow older together. We advise each other about various issues, depending on how many details of our lives we share with our List counterparts, some of whom have become telephone or real-life 2g friends. Having been on The List for more than a third of my life, for me, it is much more than a List. It is a group that accepts me as I am; a community where I feel that I belong. Most of all, it is composed of members of my 2g tribe, the one that none of us chose to be part of, where we spend our lives gravitating between its burdens and privileges, while making the best of the often unvoiced but nevertheless equally unforgettable legacy that our survivor parents bequeathed us.

Jeanette Friedman Sieradski
Taaseh Lach Chavurah – Create Your Own 'Hood

Introduction

The day after Halloween 1979, the year of the oil strikes that infuriated drivers, I drove up to B'nai Yeshurun, a large synagogue in Teaneck, where two of my babies, ages 18 months and two-and-a-half years old, were in the daycare program. I was dropping them off on the way to work as the Jewish Student Advisor at William Paterson College. As I walked my baby daughters to the entrance, I froze. Scrawled all over the yellow brick walls were swastikas and curses about the Jews.

In my life as an Orthodox Jew and then in my life as a "free" person, aka "On a Different *Derech*" (meaning I chose a path other than Orthodoxy), the only antisemitism I experienced came from secular Jews who didn't hire me when I was Orthodox, and Orthodox Jews who didn't hire me when I was secular. I, twin with a boy, was raised in a Hasidic/Haredi (ultra-Orthodox) family, although we didn't call it that back in the day. I went to an ultra-Orthodox Bais Ya'akov (Beth Jacob) girls' school in Brooklyn and had an amazing social studies and civics teacher who taught us that America was the land of the free and the home of the brave, that we were very lucky our parents found their way there, and that no one could hurt us in America. We appreciated what she taught us – along with the idea of equal rights, and the Emma Lazarus poem on the Statue of Liberty. She explained how government worked and that the Declaration of Independence and Constitution were examples of the ideals America strived to meet.

So, seeing that kind of blatant Jew-hating graffiti on the *shul* (synagogue) wall shocked me. I'd only seen stuff like that on photos from 1938 Kristallnacht and the 1940s in America. I didn't know what I was going to do, but I knew I had to do something. As a journalist by trade, though I just freelanced at the time, I took a walk around the building once my kids were inside, to see if there were more curses on the walls. While doing so, I ran into a reporter from the local news station. Clearly, the word had gotten out. She shoved a microphone in my face and asked me what I thought. I told her that my parents were Holocaust survivors, and that I was shocked, but I had to think about what I was going to do about it.

My Family History

I come from a long line of Hasidic *rebbes*, starting with the "Holy Jew", Yaakov Yitzhak Rabinowitz, and you could, in a way, call all those *rebbes* activists and community organizers. After all, they were leaders. My father, who lost his first wife and son in Auschwitz, was 100 % an activist. He served on the Jewish Rescue Committee (Vaad Hatzolah) in Hungary, where he worked with my mother's brother, Rabbi Baruch Yerachmiel Yehoshua Rabinowitz, and with Rabbi Dov Ber Weissmandl, to smuggle my mother out of the Warsaw Ghetto and bring her to Munkacs, along with other Polish Jews they tried to rescue. In America, he was a political activist and one of the leaders of World Agudath Israel Movement. My mother hosted luncheons, helped create schools, ran fundraisers, organized Nishei women (an ultra-Orthodox women's organization), hocked her jewelry to keep Camp Bnos (a girls ultra-Orthodox camp) open, while my dad helped set up *shuls*, and got communities organized in Williamsburg, Crown Heights, Borough Park and Rockland County. I grew up with *rebbes* and politicians sitting at my parents' dining room table, deciding how to rescue Jews from places like Iran in the days of the Shah, after all those years of bringing people in from the DP camps and getting matzoh to the USSR for Pesach. In other words, I grew up knowing that people who act, who do more than talk, can make a difference.

My father was born in the part of Czecholovakia that became Hungary, in a suburb of Munkacs, where his family owned the flour mill and were movers and shakers in the Munkacser *shul*. His grandfather was the Dombrader Rov (Rabbi). He had four brothers and only he and one brother survived. He was ordained at the yeshiva in Mir, was never sent to a labor camp, but was warned by a cousin (passing as a Gentile), who managed to get into the Gestapo, that he should bring his wife and child to Budapest and he would put them in a safe house. My dad didn't listen, and three days later he was in Auschwitz, where his 18-month-old son, Chaim Lazar, was ripped from his arms and sent to the gas chamber with his mother.

My mother, sister of the *Admor* (Hassidic Rabbi) of Munkacs, was born in Siedlce in Poland, where her father was the Partzever Rebbe. Almost all her brothers and brothers-in-law were Hassidic rabbis, and she was the youngest of 11. Her father died before the war, they lived in poverty, so my grandmother, Yuta, opened a pension in Warsaw on Gesia Street, where the Museum of the History of Polish Jews now sits on top of her house. She was studying at Bais Ya'akov in Krakow when the war broke out and went back home. When my uncle and my dad arranged to have them both escape in the trunk of a car, my grandmother stayed behind to protect the city's Torah scrolls, which had been piled on her dining room table. There were so many, they told me, that the table bent under their weight. She died of typhus not long after my mom escaped. My grandmother had the last formal funeral in the Warsaw ghetto.

My parents met before the war, but my uncle would not allow them to marry, telling his best friend he was not religious enough for his baby sister. When my mother ended her harrowing journey to Munkacs, my father proposed again, and she turned him down, telling him what the Germans were doing to the Jews, and that she wouldn't marry until it was over. Instead, my father married Suri Gelb, the furniture maker's daughter, and two years later he was a widower and a slave laborer, and my mom was running, in hiding. She ended up on the Kasztner Transport from Hungary and was released in Switzerland in December 1944. From there she made her way to Mandate Palestine, where she was reunited with her oldest sister and took care of the Munkacser Rebbe's children, because their mother had died of tuberculosis, and someone had to care for the five of them.

When my aunt heard my dad was still alive, she wrote him to say my mom was still alive. He wrote to her, and after a short correspondence she traveled to France where they were married. My parents travelled to America for an Agudath Israel convention, overstayed their visas, and my mother gave birth to my brother and me, the first post-war set of twins to Holocaust survivors in Bedford-Stuyvesant, Brooklyn, a badge I wear with honor.

After the UJA program for rabbis tossed my father out because he did not want to take a pulpit in South Carolina, my father went into the plastic scrap business. He would haul 50-gallon drums of scrap on his back and melt them into plastic purses that were supposed to look like they were made of pearls. He soon changed the business into making plastic tablecloths that looked like lace and were machine washable. His first factory was in West New York, the second was in Hoboken, and the big one was in Bayonne. At the same time, he would learn *Daf Yomi* (a daily page of Talmud), and help raise money for schools and *shuls*, while helping his *landsmen* build their businesses in America.

Though we lived in Brooklyn at first, my mother was a cook in New City during the summer, and then became a mikveh lady in Union City, New Jersey. My twin brother and I went to Yeshiva Hudson County, and when our younger brother was three years old, he contracted polio. Thus, we twins were among the first kids vaccinated against the disease. Once things settled down a bit, my father decided New Jersey wasn't Orthodox enough, so we moved to Crown Heights, where he was the president of the local branch of Agudath Israel and became a political activist on a grand scale. That's where the youngest in the family, our sister, was born.

My twin brother was sent to the Bobover Yeshiva, I went to Rabbi Levy's Beis Ya'akov and then to Esther Schoenfeld high school on the Lower East Side, where they taught us how to learn, not how to be puppets. I helped organize a class trip to The World's Fair, a number of Shabbatons, and we even went down to FDR Drive to welcome John Glenn back to Earth. Esther Schoenfeld was really a great high school for girls. My friends and I walked the streets of New York, especially Crown Heights, as if we owned them, and we felt like we did. And then it was time to get married.

Life Before the List

When I was 17, I was placed on the meet/meat market and my father disapproved of every guy I liked. Finally, the *shadchanim* (matchmakers) had me married off to a closeted gay Telzer yeshiva *bochur* (male student) 10 years older than I was, and whose British family was Chabad (Lubavitch). I couldn't break the engagement. Two years later, as the survivor of domestic violence with a baby, I was fighting for a *Get* (Jewish divorce). Not only was I put through a lot of grief by the ultra-Orthodox rabbinical establishment, but I was held up financially by my ex-husband to obtain my divorce. I fought and won, even against the establishment. By the time we were done, my daughter was eight, New York State had a new divorce law that said anyone who prevents an ex from remarrying doesn't get custody or community property, and Rabbi Moshe Feinstein, a major ultra-Orthodox arbiter of *Halakha* (Jewish law), ruled that women could get civil divorces without waiting for their *Gets*. By then I was in my mid-20s, and that was a big accomplishment for a kid who took on the rabbinate to free *agunot*, other "chained women" like me. I was already an activist.

I started Brooklyn College in 1965 and made it my business to go back to school while fighting for my *Get*. I switched to night school, was editor of the night school newspaper, and marched against the Vietnam war and for feminism. I met my second husband when I was president of the Student Center Board and he was hired to run SUBO, the Student Center, at night. I met him during second week of September 1970. It was love at first sight, but I didn't have my *Get*. When they tried to impose tuition on SGS (School of Graduate Studies) students, I led a campus-wide strike with Student Government that gridlocked the entire Borough of Brooklyn for almost two days. Tuition was deferred until my class graduated. I worked my way through school, first at the French Consulate on Fifth Avenue, then at Realite Magazine, then through a series of jobs, and finally at the Brooklyn Museum. My major was Art History with a minor in journalism, but when I graduated, my father refused to pay tuition for Columbia Journalism School. Instead, I started at New York University in Higher Education Administration, but after I married for the second time, I switched back to Brooklyn College to take Judaic Studies under Rabbi Dr. Schneur Lieman, a genius and fantastic teacher. While there, Yaffa Eliach, the person later responsible for the tower of photos at the United States Holocaust Memorial Museum, was my professor for the first Holocaust course taught at a unit of the City University of New York. Her little Holocaust Center in an office at the Yeshiva of Flatbush eventually became part of the Museum of Jewish Heritage – A Living Memorial to the Holocaust. But in those days, in that tiny office, working with Stella Weiselthier, Bonnie Gurewitsch and other Holocaust study pioneers, her focus was on collecting testimonies, and, as a volunteer, they trained me to interview Holocaust survivors and liberators on audio tapes. That would come in handy later, when I would interview survivors at various junctures of my activism.

In November 1975, three years after the *Get* finally came through, I married Philip Sieradski, a 2g (Second Generation) who was also a Vietnam vet. In addition to L'via (1967), the daughter of my first marriage, I had three additional children: Aviva (1977), Aliza (1978) and Daniel (1979). L'via is a registered nurse and lactation consultant and lives in Arnona in Jerusalem. Aviva is a Lubavitcher – Chabadnik who lives in Nachlaot in Jerusalem with her family. She codes, designs jewelry and is a copywriter. They left Pittsburgh about three months before the murders at the Tree of Life Synagogue. Aliza is a singer/songwriter, who was married in Jerusalem, and just moved from California to a farm in Oregon. My son Daniel is an internet pioneer who created the first Jewish blogs, he lives in Syracuse, and spent three years in Israel. He is now way left of center. Yes, I had Irish triplets, and so much for all forms of birth control.

After four years of marriage to my beloved Vietnam Vet, because of antisemitism in Teaneck, NJ, I became a 2g activist, while at the same time using the first generation of computers to contact friends everywhere, even before America On Line (now AOL) went live. So as The List of 2gs friends grew, I eventually suggested communicating via the web.

As a longtime activist I was used to stirring the pot. So, when the swastikas appeared in my town, I was not going to sit on my hands. For starters, I scheduled some Holocaust programming for the students at William Paterson College, which had not yet become pretentious enough to call itself a university. That same week, I heard about a conference sponsored by Rabbi Yitz (Irving) Greenberg's organization, Zachor, about 2gs. By that time, the *New York Times Magazine* had put Helen Epstein's book, *Children of the Holocaust,* and her story on the cover. The conference was a shrink-fest about us, not for us, but hundreds of us showed up that weekend at Hebrew Union College in Greenwich Village. Above all, the attendees discovered just how many of their friends were 2gs and they didn't know it. The conference, put together by Eva Fogelman and Bella Savrin, featured mental health professionals who dealt with Holocaust trauma in survivors and their children. It was an eye-opener, and when they tried to say we were off the wall, we proved it by standing on our seats and shouting them down. After listening to everyone but Eva tell us we were basically nuts, many of us said we came there to demand action against antisemitism and ideas on how to teach the Holocaust, as well as running rap groups to discuss our dysfunctional families. It was also at that conference I discovered that one of my mother's brothers, Yaakov Rabinowich, had escaped from Treblinka, came back to the Warsaw Ghetto, and died with a rifle in his hands, on a roof, on the first night of the Uprising, first Seder Night. He is the family hero, and we made a Haggadah in his honor.

I spent two days at that conference, and when I got home, I put an ad *The Jewish Standard* in Teaneck, inviting local 2gs to come to my home for exploratory talks about starting something useful in the community. There was no money involved. The idea was to meet other 2gs, introduce some Holocaust education into the schools, introduce Holocaust commemorations in the *shuls,* and figure out how to stop the Jew Hatred. In those days, it bubbled to the surface because gas was hard to get, and the Israelis were being blamed. According to the haters, all Jews were guilty, giving them permission to vandalize synagogues and worse.

For me, that was just not going to fly. On the advertised night, 15 people showed up at my house. One of the psychologists from the conference came to be a facilitator. I learned there were groups in other states, and certainly in New York, but I was completely unfamiliar with the "etiquette" of rap groups, and the custom of going around in a circle to have everyone say their piece. But we did that and discovered that the group was split down the middle. One half wanted rap groups and the other wanted social action. So, we split up, and from what I hear, members of that rap group are still in touch with each other. Other activists showed up that day, including Menachem Rosensaft from New York and Steve Tencer, both of whom were active in the organization of survivors from Bergen-Belsen.

What fascinated me at that first meeting in my home in Teaneck and in subsequent 2g meetings everywhere, was that people would give their names, and instead of saying I am a writer, parent, teacher, doctor, lawyer, they said "My name is___ and my mother was in Auschwitz and my father was in hiding" or similar one-line resumes of their parents in the war. It seemed strange to me, as if those were their sole credentials for existing. I was, by nature, an activist and I identified myself as such. Were they not accomplished individuals in their own right?

It turned out I founded the first 2g group in New Jersey, but I also began attending 2g meetings in New York. In 1980 we were asked to help UJA/Fed New York leader Ernest W. Michel put together something he had dreamed up when he was an inmate in Auschwitz. He wanted to bring all the survivors to Israel for a commemoration. Before we knew it, we were traveling around the country, inviting survivors and their families to come to Israel in the summer of 1981 for the World Gathering of Jewish Holocaust Survivors. It was quite something.

On the first day of the World Gathering in June 1981, my workshop was filled to the rafters. People wanted to know how to get their parents to tell their stories. And so, taking what I had learned from Yaffa and Bonnie, I interviewed Guta Tencer, Steve's mother, a woman who had given her daughter away for safekeeping in Poland and never found her again. Steve, totally devoted to his mom, was one of the earliest Second Generation activists in the greater metro New York area. I always considered him and Pnina Kaplan, both from Fair Lawn, co-founders of our group.

The person who stood out more than the others that day in Jerusalem was Syd Mandelbaum from the Five Towns, just over the New York City line. One of the pioneers of video-taping survivors, he came with his video camera and said he gave his testimony tapes to the Yale Fortunoff Archives.

My activism continued. We helped the survivors organize the American Gatherings after Israel. One in Washington, DC in 1983, and one in Philadelphia in 1985. We put together conferences and held commemorations, putting Holocaust remembrance on the Jewish calendar. Some of us went to Germany in 1985, to Bergen Belsen, President Ronald Reagan's last stop before Bitburg, to beg him not to put the wreaths on the graves of the Nazis.

Meanwhile, I had to make a living. I was working for a company owned by an Israeli that published *Right On!* and *Tiger Beat* and wrote celebrity books. He docked my pay for going to Germany. When I came back, I wrote a Rock Hudson biography, a fanzine for Miami Vice, the TV show, and articles filled with the stories of celebrities and sports stars. When that job ended, I wound up freelancing three books about New York City, reviewing night clubs, dance halls and late-night eateries. That was a wild and crazy time, where I learned that dance floors were the great equalizers between people of all races and religions. The only thing that mattered was loving to dance. Later that changed, when people began bringing knives and guns to the clubs and security became tighter than the security on El Al Airlines.

Phil and I then became editors of a prominent Jewish magazine from Canada which allowed me to interview major players from Ruth Bader Ginsburg and George Soros, to Robin Williams, Steven Spielberg, Joan Rivers, Carl Sagan, Ralph Lauren, Arik Sharon, Ehud Barak and many, many others. I was busy, but I kept in touch with my friends through a List that I had joined. It was a very interesting existence.

Life After Joining The List

Since its inception in 1995 I was on an email List of English-speaking 2gs throughout the world. I noticed there were many more women than men, and that many of them were like the people in the rap group that had broken off from the Second Generation North Jersey group. Basically, they were not interested in social action, they wanted to chat about their families and kids, and many of them expressed bitterness about how their parents created them as dysfunctional beings because of the Holocaust. I am not denying serious effects of parenting by traumatized Holocaust survivors. As I noted above, my trauma was more from the hypocrisy of what we now call Haredism (ultra-Orthodoxy) than the Holocaust, but even I had to reach a point where I made the decisions in my life and took responsibility for my own actions.

What bothered me deeply were those who refused to take responsibility for their own lives and continued to blame their parents. In addition to that, there were a few women who decided that The List was an ultimate game of the Suffering Olympics. I did not want to be part of such a competition. When I posted some complaints about Phil, who was really messed up with PTSD, sleep deprivation from running a bakery, and his mother killing him in business every day, I noticed people were playing, "Can you top that?" Ugh. We had plenty of problems with our kids, and plenty of problems with money. We lost our house at one point, and needed to start from scratch, but posting stuff like that on The List went nowhere. There was little or no emotional support. And one or two members convinced me that it was hurtful for me to post these things because it seemed others relished other people's misery and enjoyed the suffering of others. While they wanted to write about themselves, I preferred writing about action, making a difference.

The last straw on The List for me came in 1999. In 1990, I had become involved with two Jewish leaders in Sarajevo, Bosnia, who were in the middle of a vicious war between Muslims and Christians that was begun by racist dictator Slobodan Milosevic. Both were 2gs, in charge of the Jewish Community Center in the besieged town and came to America to ask for help. I brought them to a Second Generation meeting at Lincoln Square Synagogue to help them raise funds, and they were treated like dirt under people's feet. It was a disgusting display of privilege over poverty, xenophobia (who ever heard of Bosnia in those days?) and selfishness. We left, floored by the ugly behavior of our peers. Nine years later, in Kosovo, the ethnic cleansing began again in earnest, and Muslim refugees fled to Macedonia. A 2g I knew from the World Gathering who was a neighbor in Bergen County, NJ (and who thought our list was an exercise in futility), called me and said he wanted to get a group of us together, to do something about the refugees he saw on TV. I suggested we go to the refugee camp, Stankovic, in Macedonia. That was the same day as the school shooting in Columbine, Colorado, a shooting that was supposed to celebrate Hitler's birthday. He agreed, and we organized the trip with help from the Joint Distribution Committee, which had been working with Jewish leaders in Sarajevo.

Our group gathered shoes, socks, toys, medicine, sundries for women and children, collected from nearby day schools, packed it all into duffle bags and went to Macedonia. I came back, wrote about it on The List, and was accused by one member of going to Stankovic just to feed my ego and not help anyone. I quit The List, but not for the last time as I would later rejoin and leave, several times, each time the discussions blew up. Much of it had to do with the fact that I wanted to post about activism and not discuss how difficult our lives were as 2gs.

Through all this we had to make a living. Phil and I built our business, The Wordsmithy, which specialized in helping survivors write and publish their memoirs. At the same time, I was still freelancing for my local Jewish newspaper, and trying to get help for chained women. Money troubles plagued us, and finally, we lost our house in Bergen County in 2009. In 2012 we bought a giant log cabin right over the Mt. Pocono town line in Pennsylvania and began to fix it up. Phil stayed behind in New Jersey to pack us up, and I worked with the contractors. At the same time, my elderly mom got sick with kidney disease, so I went back and forth to Brooklyn, with my daughter L'via in Teaneck, to care for her. Then Phil got sick too, and the two of us switched up, going from Holy Name in Teaneck to Lutheran and Maimonides in Brooklyn.

I spent nights in the hospital convincing my mother that she was not going to die and would be present at her grandson's wedding – and we made it happen. Even she couldn't believe what mind over matter could do, and was thrilled that she was at the wedding, even though she was brought in an ambulance from the rehab center and was taken back the same day. It was one of the best days in her life, a huge victory, and she was still around when her first great-great granddaughter was born a year later.

My mother had written her own book, *Going Forward*, with a woman in Brooklyn that was published by Artscroll. It was a historical disaster. After learning the book was out of print, Phil and I rewrote and edited lots of it, added the family tree and put it out there. It sold well, and the letters my mother got from her fans enthralled her. The book I wrote with another 2g, David Gold, is called *Why Should I Care? Lessons from the Holocaust*, and it was published in 2009, taking a different approach. If anyone wants to read it, they can download it for free from academia.edu. I am very proud of that book and consider it the most important thing I ever wrote.

Meanwhile, in our new neighborhood, we were once again dealing with blatant antisemitism. We lived in Paradise Valley, in the densely wooded Pocono Mountains, about 90 miles from New York City, but because of some of the locals, it was hard to see the Paradise. The guy who was putting in our carpets asked me why we killed Jesus. The electrical contractor wanted to know why we didn't believe in God. I was introduced to Alice, an older woman who came from one of Brooklyn's oldest and staidest families who lived at the top of The Knob, the highest point in Mt. Pocono. She invited me to go to church with her one Sunday, right down the hill from me, the Innovation Church. I figured, what the heck, let me see what goes on, and I was greeted by a huge power-point slide that read: "Israelites are like washed pigs who go back to the mud, like dogs who eat their vomit." After the services I found out the church has a model of the Temple, the *Beis Hamikdash*, in another room, and the pastor accused the Jews of America for causing the Abortion Holocaust. A few weeks later, people painted swastikas on a few places in Mt. Pocono. Antisemitism without Jews.

My spirit of activism really kicked in regarding the American presidential elections. All those years teaching and writing about the Holocaust, studying HOW it happened, convinced me that we were living in dangerous times. I was certain that if Donald Trump was elected, democracy would be at stake. I went looking for the local Democrats and pleaded with them to make Holocaust Education available in the schools. They thought I was nuts and exaggerating the situation. But that was six years ago. They believe me now.

My Democratic State Representative introduced me to a woman who lives in a Homeowners Association who tried to put together a commemoration and failed. That woman introduced me to Marylou Lordi, a Roman Catholic woman, who lives 40 miles away, and helps me in every way possible. The year before the Covid-19 epidemic began, we did a county-wide commemoration on *Yom Hashoah* (Holocaust Memorial Day) that brought almost 100 people to the Mountain Center, where we displayed a huge exhibit made by a Holocaust survivor from Paramus about his experiences as a German Jew in the camps and ghettos. We got TV coverage and newspaper coverage for three days. The following year, we had to cancel because of Covid. This year Marylou and I put together a video commemoration for the county with performers from The National Yiddish Theatre and others. It's on Vimeo, but here's the link to my Dropbox, where people can watch it anytime. Those of us who worked on it are very proud of what we accomplished. https://www.dropbox.com/s/ba0z6jii7o8eftt/Monroe%20County%20Commemoration%202021.mp4?dl=0 Marylou and I decided to work toward creating a Holocaust and Human Rights Education Center for teachers. It isn't easy, but we persist.

All this took place during a period when I was not actively part of the 2g List group. I joined a few 2g groups on Facebook but they staunchly supported Trump, so I left. All they could think about was Israel, and that he was good for it. Well, I strongly disagreed, but that did not stop two of my daughters and their families from making *aliyah*. I hold my breath every time a rocket comes flying over their homes, and I hope and pray that my children, grandchildren, and great-grandchildren, will fight for human rights for everyone in the region – and especially for women's rights in Israel.

When I heard that the 2g List was being rebirthed, I joined, and as soon as I posted, the same naysayers, the *nishtfarginners* (those who didn't give credit) and Olympic sufferers came after me. The very same ones. I said "Goodbye" and haven't looked back. Until I was asked to write about my experiences for this book. I have stayed in touch privately with old members from all around the world. We visited each other in the USA, Israel, England, and Ireland. We communicate frequently and they, as individuals, have been helpful. But then again, it is hard to get together with them locally because of Covid-19. We decided that if it ever ends, I will invite a group to come for a weekend to the log cabin in the mountains. There's plenty of space to accommodate a dozen folks.

Epilogue

On September 13, 2020, Phil died a horrible, painful death, with procedures that could have been invented by Torquemada or Hitler's troops. It started the day after my daughter made *aliyah* in August, and he was dead two weeks later, a bit more than 36 hours after I brought him home to die in peace. It was almost exactly 50 years to the day we met.

During *Shiva* (week of mourning), Daniel, my son, stayed with me, and one day three friends of his who were rabbis from different denominations came to make a *Shiva* visit. They sat with him on the deck, socially distancing and all that, and chatted. I was inside. Next thing I knew, they came in and told me they had just formed a Beit Din and decided to give me *Smicha* (ordination) for all my studies in Judaism (never finished my Masters, ran out of money and time) and the Holocaust and *Agunah* work I did in the community. They gave me a test of sorts, they made a *bracha* (blessing) or two, and asked for a nice piece of paper and markers. That piece of paper now hangs in pride of place on the wall in my office, and I have the right to call myself a rabbi. I use the title judiciously. Up here, in the boonies, it helps. In Brooklyn, it's considered a joke, but it is not. It is real.

After Phil died and Marylou heard that he had been poisoned by Agent Orange, she let me know I was entitled to get a pension from the Army. Phil and I had been back and forth on it with the Veterans Administration since 1982 and I had letters to prove it. She told me to go to my local VA, and I did, bringing the medical reports of his various diseases from his doctors. After 40 years, in July 2021, the United States Army granted me a small monthly pension that will help me pay my bills – and the ability to use the G.I. Bill to further my education, if I decide to do so. Since he died, with help from Marylou and others, I now have a support group to help me rebuild my life. Only one of those helping me on a regular basis is a descendant of Holocaust survivors. Most of them aren't Jewish, although I work with Chabad rabbis in Canadensis and Scranton, helping them with local politicians and they help me get kosher food. They like me, I like them, and though they are very busy rabbis, they found time to read the *megillah* (Scroll of Esther) for us on Purim and blow the shofar. They helped with Philip's *taharah* (purification before burial). In fact, they call me the Rebbitzen (rabbi's wife) of the Poconos because they say I give them a *shem tov* (good name) up here. My response: I just laugh.

And I count my blessings. My children, all of them hundreds or thousands of miles away, are relatively healthy; they are coping with all the problems parents have, taking care of their children and their families. My married grandchildren are all happy and starting their lives in Israel and in the US. (One was married during *Shiva* and one a month or two later, both in Israel. They took my picture and put it on a stick to carry down the aisle while I watched on Zoom.) I have a nice roof over my head, Phil, on his deathbed, thanked me for making him a beautiful home and helping him be a somebody. He died on a *Motzoei Shabbos* (Saturday night) and we Zoomed his funeral, thanks to Marylou, whose son made that possible. I spend much of my time on Facebook, talking to fellow Democrats, rabbis, and people who share my political beliefs, working to affect change in America and Israel. We are living in dangerous times, and our voices count. I also stay in touch with members of The List as individuals through Facebook. I succeed by building my *chavurah* (group) of people who care about me and support me, and I care about them. Many of them are 2gs on Facebook, many of them are "reality" friends. Who am I? When I am asked to identify myself in such environments these days, I introduce myself as Jeanette Friedman, writer, reporter, publisher, and community activist. And I do that because that is mainly who I am. I still train people to interview the few survivors who are left, especially students whose schools sign up with Tova Rosenberg's Names Not Numbers program to interview survivors and make films about them. Did I get certain strengths of character and life lessons from my parents? Yes, I did. Was my life difficult because I was the older sibling in a set of twins with a boy? You betcha. So, when people said that the Holocaust ruined their lives, my story was a bit different. Because it was not the Holocaust. What I learned from my parents was how to survive and help a community survive. I wasn't messed up because of the Holocaust, I was messed up because of Judaism and its misogyny and corruption when it came to chained women (*agunot*) who could not get Jewish divorces, its tacit approval of corporal punishment, and its mixed messages while trying to find myself in the alien world called America.

So, as I have always said, since the days of yore, "It Ain't Auschwitz (yet), Keep on Truckin' ", and I intend to do so, fighting for Truth, Justice, Human Rights and Jewish Pluralism until the day I die.

by Laurie Solnik
You Can't Know What You Don't Know

I bristle at having to state "Unknown" on medical questionnaires. Medical providers assume I was adopted. No, I explain. I'm an only child of Holocaust survivors, each the only survivor of once-large families. My parents, scarred and debilitated from years in concentration camps, took their stories with them to early graves. Their heavy cigarette habits and lingering heartbreaks hastened their coronaries, leaving me with no parents, siblings, aunts, uncles, or grandparents, only far-away, distant cousins and one elderly great-aunt. Everyone else in my family was murdered, so I can't tell you if there was any diabetes or cancer.

I'm acutely aware that I was the very last, most fragile link in a formerly solid chain of generations of Polish Jews going back hundreds of years. They left no trace of their existence, only that which the Nazis couldn't steal or kill off – their DNA, now residing in my body, and those of my children and their children.

My parents never spoke of what they endured in the Holocaust. A village of synagogue women and moms-of-friends guided me toward adulthood but couldn't fill in the gaps of my family's missing story. So, in the late '90s, when I learned of an online, private discussion list for children of Holocaust survivors, I thought maybe I could glean a nugget or two of insight. Little did I know that, by joining, I would ultimately find myself.

What I Didn't Know Until Later

My father and his family hailed from the town of Chmielnik in south central Poland. As far as I (and DNA tests) can tell, they had settled in the area hundreds of years before. My father was the only son among a multitude of daughters and, along with his older brother-in-law, was being groomed to enter the family business, which included a lumber yard and a sawmill.

The urban branch of his family lived in the big city of Lodz, some one hundred miles to the north. As the young people of Chmielnik came of age, some migrated to Lodz, lodging there with extended family while they honed a trade or pursued a *shidduch* (marriage match), returning to Chmielnik to raise families of their own.

A generation or two earlier, this Lodz branch of my family, also named Solnik, had become electricians when they received one of Poland's first contracts to extend power lines into rural areas. The city dwelling Solniks offered their country bumpkin Chmielniker relatives first dibs on electrification. The Chmielnikers initially declined, not trusting either the technology or the technicians, or both. A family feud ensued and, while the lumber mill was eventually electrified, the rift between progressive urban and conservative rural inclinations continued.

My mother's small *shtetl* (village) of Nowy Korczyn, also in south central Poland, was a verdant but poor trading hamlet originally settled in 1258. Over the centuries, it was burned, pillaged, and flooded repeatedly until it lost its charter entirely in 1860 and settled into backwater obscurity. My mother was a middle child whose older sisters helped care for their younger siblings, leaving my mother free to dream of a future she knew could only exist in her imagination. One of the *shtetl's* clergy, *der rebbe* (the rabbi) Epshteyn, was a grizzled old man with a long, white beard and an even longer black coat. He was a wise *rebbe* who, foreseeing trouble ahead in Europe, had fled to America well before the war, along with some of his followers. I am eternally grateful for his prescience.

My mother and father were acquainted before the war because my mother played with my father's younger sisters when visiting the markets of nearby Chmielnik. But as the daughter of a poor baker, she never could have aspired to such a lofty match. The war, however, was the great equalizer, robbing its survivors of wealth, family, status, and expectations.

After liberation from their respective concentration camps, each of my parents made their way back to their homes, only to find them destroyed or otherwise occupied. During this time, while waiting to see if any family members might also stagger back (none did), my parents became a couple. In 1946, with the postwar Kielce *pogrom* (organized massacres) breaking out nearby, the area wasn't safe for returning Jews, so my parents headed to the American sector of Berlin for security and opportunity.

My father traveled first to scout out living options and found a modest attic room. Before he could send for my mother, he developed a festering, oozing infection on the bridge of his nose where his glasses, which he learned to never remove, had rubbed his skin raw. Realizing in the camps that his poor eyesight would have been a death sentence, my father slept with his glasses on, a habit he continued after liberation. By the time my mother found him, a high fever and delirium had set in. Without identification papers or funds, and with an aversion to seeking medical treatment, my mother surgically cut, cleaned, and stitched the wound herself, nursing my father back to health.

Soon they were joined in the attic room by my father's second cousin from Lodz, Chanaleh, and her second husband, Yosseleh. Having only four in a room must have felt quite luxurious after years of squeezing into Nazi barracks. They lived quiet, undocumented lives under the radar while stealthily operating a successful black-market smuggling operation. My father would obtain goods from the Americans, load up my mother with suitcases of merchandise and multiple layers of clothing, then put her on a train back to Poland where others would offload the goods and my mother would return with cash. They did this for two years, saving their money for their as yet undetermined future.

Through documents I obtained from the United States Holocaust Memorial Museum in Washington, DC where I live, I learned that my mother filled out multiple applications with the United Nations International Refugee Resettlement Agency (UNIRRA), requesting resettlement in Palestine or the United States or anywhere that wasn't Europe, using variations of her birth name, her married name and even her nickname.

When *der rebbe* Epshtyn learned that only 67 of his *shtetl's* 2,600 Jews had survived the Holocaust, he actively worked to secure their resettlement. Additionally, my mother recalled she had an aunt who had immigrated to New Jersey at the end of the 19th century. My mother hired an American G.I. to write to this aunt, whom she had only met once as a child on the aunt's return visit to Poland in 1932, introducing herself as one of the many children who had posed for a formal family photo commissioned by the aunt during that visit. I have that photo today, the only image left of my mother's once large, extended family. I can identify my mother and the visiting aunt, but not the others in the photo. I don't even know their names.

"I am not sure if you remember me," my mother wrote to her aunt from post-war Germany. "But I'm the only one left. I have a husband now and we'd like to go to Palestine. If you can send us some money, we promise to repay you as quickly as we can."

With the help of *der rebbe* Epshteyn and his followers, the International Red Cross, the UNIRRA, and the New Jersey aunt who was thrilled to learn that anyone in her family had survived at all, my parents began their new lives in America. I was born in New Jersey in 1953, after years of primitive fertility treatments aimed at preventing my mother's unstable womb from continuing to miscarry.

What is Family Anyway?

I didn't know how much I didn't know, until I began to realize that many of the people I'd thought of as my extended family weren't related to me at all. Nor were they even longtime family friends. Most were a ragtag assortment of Holocaust survivors who became attached to my parents either en route to their new, post-war life in America, or shortly after their arrival. I didn't know that my Uncle Natan and Tante (aunt) Yadjeh weren't my parents' actual siblings, or that their children weren't my real cousins. How could I know? We were together every holiday, in and out of each other's homes on weekends and in summers, cooking the same foods, speaking the same dialect, angered at the same triggers.

It would start off in Yiddish, which we kids understood and spoke, with the adults sitting around the table chatting pleasantly enough. Yiddish phrases beginning with *in der heim* ("back home") were usually followed by a trip down memory lane of life before Hitler. After a round or two, someone would invariably switch to *ober in der krieg* or *in der milchumeh* ("but during the *war*") and then the tone would shift, along with the language being spoken.

Right on cue, Uncle Natan would explode, claiming the grand prize in the hierarchy of suffering. "You think YOU had it bad? I had it MUCH worse!" This was the signal for Tante Yadjeh to retreat to the kitchen. The children would scatter to the bedrooms and the house would reverberate with the booming sounds of every high-pointed Scrabble letter in the Polish language. The words were a mystery to us children, but their tone was clear. When the adults were spent and the children sleepy, the evening and its drama would end, only to be repeated next time and the time after, in the same order.

Didn't everybody's gatherings start and end this way? Doesn't every adult have numbers tattooed onto their left forearms? Would I get my numbers, too, when I grew up? Do other kids' dads also wake up screaming at night? Is it normal for a child to sit in a darkened kitchen sharing a pot of warm milk with a parent who can't sleep? Are grandparents real? Nobody I knew had any. Do they just exist on TV?

My mother's New Jersey aunt, known to me simply as Tante, wanted nothing to do with the pseudo-family my parents had collected among their fellow survivors. Tante, a quiet older woman, particularly disliked Uncle Natan, who was bombastic. This seemed like an ordinary personality conflict until I overheard something about stealing gold teeth from cadavers as he pulled them from the gas chambers and delivered them to the crematoria.

"Why should the Nazis get everything?" he said. My parents never judged. Tante did.

On each minor Jewish holiday, in appreciation for the resettlement help, my father, mother and I would dress up in our fancy best to pay homage to (and leave a donation for) *der rebbe* Epshtyn and his followers, all of whom could fit around the long, white-clothed table that took up most of his cramped, Lower East Side apartment. I was always the only child in attendance. I'd squeeze in with my clean-shaven father at the table filled with bearded, black-hatted men, and we'd bang our palms on the tabletop to the rhythm of *niggunim* (wordless melodies). It was joyful and I loved my perch on my father's lap.

Until I was nine years old. Then, for reasons never explained to me, I was banished to the kitchen with the women. All they did was gossip, stir pots of food, and speak of *in der heim*. They never mentioned *in der krieg*, most having fled before the war. Once, on our way out, during lingering goodbyes in the long, narrow apartment building hallway, I leaned against the far wall near the elevator to wait for my mother. *Rebbe* Epshtyn stepped into the hallway at one point but stopped suddenly when he saw me. Everyone hushed up, but *der rebbe* didn't proceed. All eyes slowly turned toward me, though I didn't know why. Then, as if a lightbulb turned on in my mother's brain, she grabbed me rather roughly and jerked me to her side of the hallway so that *der rebbe* could continue walking without having to pass between two women. This was the environment in which my parents and their parents had been raised. These visits to *der rebbe,* lacking explanation or context, were my only window into their lost world.

I was the cause of The Big Rift of our pseudo-family that year. My mother figured that, if I could be considered a woman at that age, I'd better learn some life skills. Skills? I'd never done any chores and I certainly didn't know my way around responsibility. Clothing mysteriously got cleaned and put away, meals cooked, dishes washed, and beds made, with no particular effort on my part. My only job until then was to be happy. This expectation was a particular burden when I got upset over, say, a broken doll or a missed playdate. "After all your parents went through," chided my pseudo-cousins, "You're crying over a doll? A **DOLL**?" In the hierarchy of suffering, my trauma was irrelevant.

So that summer, my mother sent me off to sleep-away camp halfway across the country. It was a music camp that a schoolmate had attended the year before. My mother was intent on molding me into a proper American. What could go wrong?

"You're sending away your only child?" demanded Uncle Natan. "To a *camp*? Didn't you have enough of camps during the war? How could you do this to your own child?!!!" And then he spit out a slew of words in Polish as he gathered up his family and stormed out. Thus ended our cozy, extended fake-family experiment. But I liked the summer camp. The irony of my getting the junior division's "Most Improved Camper" award at the end of the summer was, of course, lost on me.

I'll never know whether my enrollment in Hebrew School that fall was in response to Uncle Natan's religious virtue signaling or my parents' discovery that I had tasted bacon at music camp. Beginning that school year, three times a week I trudged to the nearby Conservative synagogue for afterschool lessons in a language that looked, but didn't sound, like the Yiddish newspapers my parents read. I didn't much like Hebrew School, but my mother was determined that I have an American-style Bat Mitzvah with a party to which she could invite all her friends, American and immigrant alike.

Then, exactly one month before my Bat Mitzvah, in the middle of a frigid February night, after painting the kitchen walls in preparation for out-of-town guests who might come to the house, my mother unexpectedly dropped dead. My father, never one for words anyway, sobbed uncontrollably before settling into the silence that enveloped him for the dozen years he had left. The door to any family history was nailed as tightly shut as their coffins.

One Door Closes, Another Opens

My mother was pronounced dead just before 3:00 am, following my father's unsuccessful efforts to revive her and my own fruitless call to 911 in my little girl voice. The funeral home took her body away before dawn to prepare it for burial before the Sabbath began that same evening. My father sat in the kitchen in a catatonic trance, so I thumbed through my mother's little black address book trying to figure out who to notify. I selected the two biggest *yentas* (gossipers) I could find among my mother's friends and called them just before dawn – one a survivor, the other an American, knowing the news would then spread like wildfire.

It seemed my mother hadn't felt well all week, attributing her growing indigestion to strong coffee and her self-induced anxiety over hosting my upcoming Bat Mitzvah. But she didn't seek medical attention, nor did my father on her behalf. They avoided doctors in general, though they always ensured I had ample care. My mother's years in Bergen Belsen and Dachau, and my father's years in Theresienstadt and Buchenwald, taught them to never, ever, display frailty. Better to tough it out. Sick inmates didn't last.

The funeral was conducted at 11:00 am that same morning, a mere eight hours after her death. My mother had carefully cultivated numerous social circles among the Americans she so admired, and she had many survivor friends who respected her ability to cultivate those Americans, given her thick European accent. At least 200 people gathered at her graveside that bleak, icy morning when a chartered bus carrying *der rebbe* Epshtyn and his followers pulled up. Our local rabbi had already begun the graveside service when all eyes turned to the parade of bearded men in long black coats, curled sidelocks swaying in unison as they trudged toward the open hole in front of my mother's plain pine casket. The crowd parted for them, *der rebbe* himself in the lead. The local rabbi, a younger, American fellow, stepped aside and *der rebbe* began the funeral anew, this time entirely in Yiddish. Then *der rebbe* and his entourage boarded the bus for their return home in time for the Sabbath. I never saw them again.

I was given the option of cancelling or rescheduling my Bat Mitzvah. The pink, flowery invitations I had painstakingly hand addressed had not yet been mailed. The party, of course, was cancelled but I knew I had to go through with the ceremony as planned. So, thirty days after my mother's death, I stood on our synagogue's *bima* (raised podium) and looked out at the same 200 people who had attended her funeral. Even without *der rebbe* and his flock, my Bat Mitzvah service felt like Funeral, Part Two. Leading that service was the hardest thing I've ever done in my life. My mother would have been proud. I showed no frailty. I toughed it out. I lasted.

Knowing he was ill prepared to raise a teenage daughter on his own in the turbulent 1960s, my newly widowed father soon reached out to his first cousin, Sali, a fellow Holocaust survivor who had resettled in Israel. That we had a close cousin at all was news to me, although I did recall those mysterious thin, blue, folded aerograms written in Yiddish cursive that occasionally arrived in our mailbox. Sali lived in Tel Aviv, where she and her husband were raising two sons who were conveniently close to my age. I was shipped off to visit them every summer after that for a healthy dose of *Yiddishkeit*, some pseudo-mothering, plenty of familiar foods and zero chance of bacon.

I loved those summers, running with my newly discovered boy cousins and their glorious gang of irreverent *sabras* (native born Israelis), none of whom had any interest in the dead past. Indeed, they scorned it and actively discouraged any discussion of life before 1948. Not once did I hear, "*In der heim.*" I was learning to straddle between worlds – immigrant,

American, observant, secular, gentile, and now Israeli. There was breadth to my upbringing, but little depth.

Finding The List

Years passed. Then decades. I went to college, backpacked through Europe while attempting unsuccessfully to avoid Germany, married, raised two sons, built a respectable career, divorced and was a happy empty nester living a charmed, urban life when I met George and Mark, a couple who lived across the park. We became regular dog-walking acquaintances, even though my large Rottweiler (my ex's breed choice) was wary of their three tiny terriers. During one walk, George mentioned, as an aside to a completely different story, that he was a child of Holocaust survivors. I stopped in my tracks to pepper him with questions. I learned his parents were from Poland. The same province in Poland. In fact, neighboring towns. George could even speak Yiddish. I felt like I'd just discovered a new pseudo-cousin.

In due time George told me about a private email discussion group for children of Holocaust survivors, known simply as The List. While internal exchanges were supposed to be confidential, George began to share with me some of the frustration he felt when List topics of great importance to him devolved into petty arguments among other members. It triggered in me an unexpectedly warm recollection of the immigrant conversations of my childhood, arguments and all, and I knew I wanted in.

Introductions were made and I was admitted to The List in the late 1990s, initially lurking to get a feel for the tone and rhythm of the group. Plus, I was curious to learn details of the various and ongoing List dramas which had so irritated George. Instead, that first morning I logged in as a member, all I saw were dozens of postings from all over the world, each with the subject line, "Happy Birthday, Marty!"

I scrolled down to a Canadian named Harvey, one of Marty's well-wishers, and recognized his surname from my Bat Mitzvah guest list more than four decades earlier. I remembered having written that name and address on one of those pink, flowery invitation that never got mailed in the aftermath of my mother's death. The family were *landsman* (fellow countrymen) of my father who had settled in Toronto after the war. I vaguely recalled having visited Harvey's home on the way back from music camp one summer, though Harvey, being a few years older, may not have been there. The survivor world can be pretty small.

It seemed like a genial enough email group of perhaps 60 or so members at its height. We were a microcosm, this generation born to survivors who'd been scattered across the world. We were an English-speaking group of mostly Americans and Israelis, with a smattering of Australians, Canadians, Brits, Irish, French, Germans and more, all of us with an inherited connection to the most awful genocide in history. Some had been born in displaced persons camps while their parents awaited resettlement. Others were the product of one survivor parent but not the other. Some List members, to my surprise, weren't raised Jewish at all, their parents having shed all allegiance to a faith they felt had abandoned them. Many, like me, maintained a level of obligatory observance that didn't match our actual belief. Others were devout, either by choice or by habit.

"How can you believe in God after all that happened in the Holocaust?" I once asked a friend who was also a child of Holocaust survivors, though not a member of The List. "Where were all God's miracles when our parents needed them?" I demanded.

"Look in the mirror," he said gently. "There's the miracle. You weren't supposed to have been born at all. The fact that you exist today *is* the miracle." This revelation, coming just as I was joining The List, totally shifted my paradigm, propelling me from embittered skeptic to triumphant miracle in what seemed like 60 seconds flat.

The List's online conversations could be as passionate and intense as any I'd heard in my childhood, but now they were occurring in my adulthood, where I could actually process them. As I began to add my thoughts to various threads being discussed, I could see themes emerging. Each thread had its own subject line, some as benign as favorite recipes, others as frightening as worst nightmares. There were some very angry List members, some timid ones, some sensible ones, a couple of comedians and a few lurkers. Everyone who posted had a story and every story garnered comments. Some would pour their hearts out, others shared only snippets of their past and current feelings, still others focused on their futures. There were a fair number of nurturers on The List who had gravitated toward various healing professions. Accomplished authors, scientists, musicians, educators, and historians abounded, reflecting not just the talents imbedded in their DNA but a drive to live and thrive and accomplish despite their inherited trauma.

The List topic that most captivated me was guilt. Jewish guilt. Survivor guilt. Stifled guilt. Manipulative guilt. Guilt can focus our attention on the feelings of others and often we assuage our guilt by denying our own feelings. The List was a place to explore those feelings, a private place made safe by a series of volunteer administrators who moderated the discussions with sensitivity. Well, most of the time. When topics devolved, some List members would quit in a huff, only to rejoin after they'd calmed down.

Others would lurk for a while, then disappear. New members would pop up, triggering an occasional need for the veterans to retell their own stories, often with a fresh insight that comes from deep reflection over time. Whenever there was a bus bombing or other violence in Israel, The List would come alive with concern for those in harm's way. It was therapeutic for me to care about these strangers and to feel equally cared about by them.

I was surprised at how important The List was becoming to me when, on a sunny morning on September 11, 2001, I arrived at my top floor office located directly across the Potomac River from the Pentagon. The World Trade Center had just been hit by a hijacked airplane and my colleagues were glued to the television in an office that had a panoramic view of the city and its surrounding area. As we watched the TV with horror, one of my colleagues nudged me and pointed out the window across the river toward the Pentagon, asking "What was that?" A large plume of smoke was rising into the air across the river when he added, "I thought that plane came in kind of low."

I didn't see the plane, just the huge cloud of smoke it created on impact. The next 10 minutes were among the oddest I'd ever experienced, a strange juxtaposition of watching the World Trade Center in flames on the TV while the Pentagon went up in smoke before our very eyes just across the river. We honestly didn't believe what our own eyes were seeing out that window because CNN had not yet reported the Pentagon hit. I tried calling my sons, one of whom lived in New York City, but I couldn't get through. When a headline finally scrolled across the TV screen confirming the Pentagon attack, we were told to evacuate the building. I unsuccessfully tried to reach my sons again, then – for reasons I still can't fathom – I shot off a quick email to The List before heading into a crowded stairwell for the 10-flight walk down to the chaos in the streets.

In normal times, fire drills were held regularly. We all knew to use the stairs and meet at a designated location outside the building so that Ron from Administration could check us off his fire drill list. Then we typically went right back to work. But when I exited the building that fateful morning and looked out to my right, I saw flames shooting skyward from the far side of the Pentagon. Sirens wailed throughout the city. A car pulled up and its driver lowered the windows and raised the volume on the radio for the gathered crowd. This was how we learned the second World Trade Center tower had fallen and that there was still one highjacked plane in mid-air, unaccounted for but presumed to be heading toward Washington. I realized then that, not only would I not be going back to work that morning, but that the world as I knew it had changed forever.

The next days and weeks were awful. Police checkpoints now separated my home from my office and, while I should have felt comforted by the armed presence, it felt more like an occupation. Was I subconsciously channeling my parents' ghetto confinements, even though the situations were completely different? I felt the same gut punch nearly two decades later when, on January 6, 2021, the National Guard was called to my neighborhood following the failed insurrection at the US Capitol, 12 blocks away. A six-mile wall of seven-foot-tall fencing topped with razor wire went up overnight around the Capitol, effectively blocking my neighborhood from the rest of the city for months. Tourists disappeared, replaced by thousands of uniformed soldiers with automatic weapons, riot shields, bulky bullet-proof vests, and idling Humvees. I reached out to The List, as I also had done at the beginning of the Covid pandemic lockdowns, when mental images of Anne Frank in hiding crept into my subconscious, despite fully realizing the situations were completely different. List members were incredibly helpful to me, particularly Paula from Canada who had worked with aging survivors. She assured me that elderly survivors were taking the lockdown well because, after all, nobody was trying to kill them.

Why had The List become so important to me? Why did I reach for it in times of distress? What did I expect anyone on The List to do? I still don't fully understand, but in addition to great comfort, The List gave me reasons to look things up, to question my own assumptions, to take advantage of my new-ish ability to conduct research online. It helped me as I developed a need to know where my family was from, where and how their families were murdered, what my parents endured and more. Over the years, this developing curiosity also led me to reach out to some folks from my childhood pseudo-family with whom I'd lost touch (or who had abandoned me?) after my mother's death.

One such family consisted of parents Chanka and Shaul, their teenage daughter, Judy, and younger son, Zanny. (I never knew if Zanny was his real name or a nickname, butT it was oddly pronounced Zenny.) They owned a chicken farm in Vineland, NJ, and visiting them was always a treat. "Look!" my mother would exclaim on the traffic-free country roads. "It's President Kennedy's highway!" And we would pretend we were the VIPs for whom the road had been cleared.

During one such visit, Chanka took me aside and whispered, "You know, your mother and I were in the camps together." My nine-year-old self was not impressed, having just spent a whole summer at music camp, myself. No context was offered, and I didn't ask. Instead, Zanny and I would hop into his family's old pickup truck, with pre-teen Zanny at the wheel using a large, wooden block strapped to his foot to reach the gas pedal and clutch, and off we'd drive to the chicken coops at the other end of their property. The chickens were a wonder to me, as was the mechanized conveyer belt that automatically sorted their eggs into cartons by size and weight. I had sweet memories of us city folks visiting our country 'kin,' where my parents seemed so happy and, unlike our visits with Uncle Natan, nobody ever slammed a palm on a table or stormed out in anger.

My father's second cousin Chanaleh, with whom my parents had shared the attic room in Berlin after liberation, was a *farbisseneh* (bitter) character. Now on her third husband, Chanaleh had seen her first husband and young daughter shot to death in front of her during the SS liquidation of the Lodz ghetto. Her only surviving son, Henyek, having endured Auschwitz and later immigrated to America with his young bride, Toby, became a beloved younger brother figure to my father. Henyek generously shared with me his recollections of life before, during, and after Auschwitz, but this was his history, not that of my parents. Until, that is, he and Toby were interviewed for a book about their Holocaust experiences.

The book, called Sarah's Children by Suzan E. Hagstrom, described how five siblings from Chmielnik managed to defy odds by surviving intact. Around the time the book came out, I ran into Shaul and Chanka on a flight to Israel. Though he had aged, Shaul's bushy brown eyebrows were unmistakable. By now they had sold the chicken farm. He and Chanka had also been interviewed for Sarah's Children. In reading that book, a treasure trove of random factoids from my childhood began to make some sense.

My mother bore deep scars on the backs of both her legs. Whenever I would ask about them, she would dismiss my questions with a wave. "It's nothing," she would say. "Just some oil spilled," and she would quickly change the subject. In reading Sarah's Children, I learned about the German munitions factory known as Hasag *lager* (camp), where my mother was a slave laborer. I recognized the name from my childhood but knew it only as a prelude to curses in Polish. Now I learned about its manufacturing process. Twenty-four hours a day, seven days a week, slave laborers would hoist giant, heavy bars of metal into one end of the machinery while other workers were positioned at the opposite end of the machinery to quickly pack the completed bullets into boxes as they were spit out. In between, still other workers would have to continually lubricate every part of the machine while it was in operation. Occasionally, noted the book's author, boiling oil would spurt back out at the lubricators, causing them disfiguring burns.

I quizzed my father's Israeli Cousin Sali, who I learned had also worked alongside my mother in Hasag *lager*. I asked how they managed to survive, fearing deep down that, as young women, they might have been sexually exploited by their captors.

"No, we made bullets," Sali explained before digressing into her own experiences. I didn't initially grasp the Hebrew word *neshek* (ammunition) and certainly didn't know its Yiddish equivalent. "You know," Sali insisted in frustration, forming one hand into a gun shape while tapping its palm with the other, saying "Little balls, we made little balls." I remained blank until she pointed toward me and said, "Boom, boom." Oh.

I read books. I watched movies and documentaries. As survivors' sagas got documented by Stephen Spielberg's Shoah Project, I mourned my inability to hear my parents' stories from their own mouths. I chatted up every Holocaust survivor I came across, including George's parents after we connected. The opening of the US Holocaust Memorial Museum within walking distance of my home in Washington, DC, became an informational lifeline. But it was The List that offered me a safety net on the emotional roller coaster of uncovering my family's story.

Meeting The List

I don't remember when my participation in The List visits began. Some members of the Israeli contingent already knew each other, connected by favorable geography and loose professional or personal ties. The next largest cluster of List members lived in the New York City area and, when an in-person gathering was suggested, I was more than happy to travel to meet them. I felt warmly welcomed, as if we'd always been pseudo-family, though this time nobody had cleared "President Kennedy's highway" for my travel. Pretty soon, I was meeting up with List members who visited DC for a conference or event, and I began looking up other List members when I traveled to their locations, deepening our individual as well as group ties.

My next List milestone was meeting the Israeli contingent. I had been visiting my Israeli family about every two years throughout my adulthood, so expanding my social circles during these trips seemed like a logical step. We first met as a group at a café in Azrieli, a large shopping mall in Tel Aviv. Though that meeting, in a crowded public space, didn't have the *haimish* (homey) feel of the New York in-home gatherings, I was thrilled to finally meet so many of the individuals I'd grown to admire, now gathered around several bistro tables. Subsequent Israeli contingent meetings occurred in people's homes, and pretty soon I was getting together with individual Israeli List members as our friendships expanded further.

The Pilgrimage

During one of the New York contingent's gatherings, a List member named Betty shared with us details of her recent, life-changing trip back to Poland with her elderly, survivor mother. Visiting Poland wasn't high on my priority list at that point. The March of the Living, an annual gathering of survivors and their descendants at Auschwitz, seemed way too large, and I didn't have survivors to accompany me. I was loathe to step foot in any of the actual camps my parents had been held in, having studiously avoided visiting Dachau during my college backpacking adventure. Now I envied those who still had parents with whom to explore roots and history. I was honored to hear Betty's deeply personal story.

George, who had introduced me to The List, also shared with me details of the Poland trip he had taken with his parents. It was strange and yet familiar to watch film after film of someone else's travelogue, and I was enormously grateful to George and his parents for letting me view their very intimate journey. Still, I couldn't envision how such a journey could unfold for me, averse as I was to group tours and lacking survivor parents to join me.

A couple of years later, Betty sent me a flyer promoting an upcoming United Synagogue Youth (USY) Alumni Jewish Heritage Tour to Poland. I was about to discard it when I noticed the trip was to be led by a then well-regarded Holocaust educator who had been my youth group advisor 45 years earlier. The concentration camps listed on the itinerary were, thankfully, not the exact ones my parents had been held in. If ever a proverbial light was meant to illuminate the dark emptiness of my family's story, this trip could be it. Despite my dislike of buses and schedules, I signed up.

I arrived in Warsaw on a warm, late June day in 2013, along with 35 others on our tour. Five of us were children of Holocaust survivors, though I was the only List member. Even the second generation of the survivor world can be quite small. Our itinerary covered several concentration camps, many neglected Jewish cemeteries and a handful of restored (but otherwise unused) synagogues. What I didn't know until I arrived at our last camp, Treblinka, was that this was the exact final destination for the Jews from both of my parents' towns. This was no work camp. It was a killing factory.

Listed there, in bold black lettering on a wall displaying the names of communities whose inhabitants were murdered there, were my father's town of Chmielnik and my mother's hamlet of Nowy Korczyn. This was where all my grandparents, aunts, uncles and extended family were sent following the Nazi roundups of their ghettos. This was where they disembarked from packed cattle cars. This was where they were made to strip naked and were driven directly into the gas chambers. Might it have been Uncle Natan plucking out their gold teeth before taking their bodies to the crematoria?

It was a lot to unpack, but I knew The List would be there for me, and they were. How had my parents avoided the fate that befell their families? I'd learned from others that my father and his brother-in-law had jumped from their transport after plying their Ukranian guards with bottles of vodka, only to be caught in the Polish countryside a few days later. The brother-in-law, not heeding an order to halt, was shot dead on the spot. My father was placed on a subsequent transport that took him elsewhere. I don't know what he did in Theresienstadt or why he was transferred to Buchenwald. I just know he was liberated from there in early April 1945.

My mother maintained that she wasn't at home for the roundup, that she had gone to a friend's farm. This, I came to understand, was her way of telling me she had run away to hide. In my early research, I came across a compilation of memories gathered by a gentile Belgian woman who had returned to her Polish grandparents' farm in the Nowy Korzcyn area seeking to document their wartime recollections, including any contact they'd had with Jews. Among the one-or two-word recollections written on the list was my mother's nickname. Just her nickname, nothing else. If my mother had, indeed, found shelter there, how did she wind up Hasag *lager*? How is it that she was liberated from Dachau, also in April 1945?

I've pieced together enough for now because I'm still processing what I've learned, and still learning about what I've processed. While my family's history will remain incomplete, I could never have tackled this project without The List's emotional support and encouragement as I mined my own memories, collected documents, read, questioned others and learned.

I can now accept that my existence is, indeed, a miracle. But did it come at too high a price? I look at Tante's 1932 family portrait, now restored, enlarged, framed. and displayed in my home. The haunting eyes of my soon-to-be slaughtered family gaze back at me and I think, no. The price was too high.

But then I look into the innocent eyes of my five young grandchildren who share my murdered family's DNA and I think, "Hmmph. Take THAT, Hitler!"

Dr. Ruth Samuel Tenenholtz
We Are Family: A Journey with the 2G Discussion List

Introduction

I was born in 1946, and my parents named me Bela Betsie Margriet, after two aunts murdered in Sobibor, and a little royal princess born in Canada during WWII. In a way, my name is my story in a nutshell.

I was born in the Netherlands, a country where almost all the survivors were people who had managed to avoid being caught in the Nazi net by going into hiding, whether in the Netherlands themselves, or somewhere abroad, whether living with false identity papers, or living in cellars and attics, secreted away, and protected by good Dutchmen, far from the public eye. The "Surviving Remnant" (*She'erit Hapletah*) in the Netherlands suffered from collective survivor guilt on such a scale that they denied that they had suffered at all. The hierarchy of suffering meant that unless you were dead, survived a camp, escaped from a train, you had not gone through anything, and surviving was not something to be proud of.

This was the milieu in which I grew up, and for the first decade of my life I knew nothing of my parents' history. Even my two older sisters were survivors, but all were tight-lipped, and stories were few and far between. I worked out my own explanations for everything that was strange in our home, and I did not ask whether my hypothesis was correct. The fact that we were the only surviving Jewish family in the village also made it impossible to compare our family's way of life to that of the surroundings, and so everything that was uncomfortable, secret, covered in cobwebs of denial, I put down to our Jewishness.

Before I Was Born

Before I was born, there were 140,000 Jews in the Netherlands, out of a population of about 12 million. In other words, about 1 % of all the Dutch population was Jewish. Half of the Jews lived in Amsterdam, comprising 10 % of the population there. The Jews called Amsterdam *Mokum* – "**the place**" (in Hebrew), perhaps the safe place, and this denotation entered the Dutch language as a loanword. The rest of the Jewish community was dispersed throughout the rest of the country. To differentiate the small communities of Jews living in the rural areas from those in Mokum, they were called the Jews of the *Mediene*, the "countryside" in Hebrew, but what it really meant was that those Jews lived in the boondocks, and that is where I came from.

Before the war, the village where I was born had barely 10 men for the weekly services, and dispersed throughout the hamlets of the municipality, there were fewer than fifty Jews. My mother came for another small village, but they boasted a larger Jewish community. They even had a Jewish theatre club. In general, because of their small numbers, the Jews of the *Mediene* were well integrated in the social fabric of the area, and perhaps the major difference was that Jews observed the Sabbath, while the Christians went to church on Sunday. If the Jews were farmers, their fields would be silent on their day of rest. But that was before I was born.

Another thing I did not experience was that our community had originally been founded by my great-grandfather, who moved there, got married, and raised a large family with many sons. When the sons came of age, they took (Jewish) wives from neighboring villages, and together, they dreamed of building a dynasty in the village. The Jews tended to live in close proximity to each other, clustered around the synagogue, kosher butchers, and their own shops, so that the villages of the *Mediene* had streets with a Jewish ambience, just as *Mokum* did. The Jews of the *Mediene* may not have been great Torah scholars, but they observed the commandments and lived according to the Jewish tradition.

None of those Jewish streets survived the war, nor did most of the Jews who had settled there with dreams of a great future, yet I never knew of their existence. It has taken me years to know the terrible loss my parents suffered as a result of the persecution of the Jews. My fingers and toes are not enough to count their number. My father lost five aunts and uncles, their spouses and offspring, his cousins. Because of Jewish tradition to name new babies after their grandparents, quite a few of his murdered cousins bore the same name as he did, and at least one bore the same name as his little daughter. My father's elderly parents and younger sister were murdered too. Most of these relatives perished in Sobibor, some in Auschwitz, and a few died in the snow of the death marches toward the end of the war. My mother lost at least seven aunts and uncles, their spouses, and offspring. Several bore the same name as she did. They also perished in Sobibor, Auschwitz, and the death marches, sometimes on the same day as my father's relatives. I count approximately fifty people, but there may have been more.

Perhaps not quite as many, but certainly devastating enough to change the survivors of the catastrophe forever.

My parents lived through the war by going into hiding. They actually remained in the village, and spent the entire war there, but for over two years, they lived in places not always suitable for human habitation. They spent days and nights in the bell tower of the Dutch Reform Church; lived much of the time behind the bakery of the Scheffer family, where a trap-door existed so they could literally go underground during the frequent house searches that the Germans carried out to look for contraband, hidden radios, weapons, Jews, and other forbidden things. Yes things, not people. The Scheffer family had all those, and they kept the resistance's weapons and other equipment hidden under the trapdoor. My parents slid down there when danger came too close.

They had been given false identity papers by the underground, and my father had grown a moustache which he dyed red, but still, they never actually went outside unless they were fleeing to another address. First of all, they were too well known around the village, and second, going outside also endangered the rescuers. While their main hiding place was with the Scheffer family, from time to time, they had to return to the church which had orchestrated their rescue in the first place. The church was across the street. After dark, when the curfew had gone into effect, the 10-year-old son of the verger would shepherd them across. He would check that the street was deserted, and then my mother and father ran for the safety of the church.

Shortly before my parents disappeared from sight, they handed over their two daughters to the resistance. It was considered better if they did not know where their children were, in case they were picked up and tortured. That is what they thought. If they did not know, they could not give the families that were sheltering their children away.

Miraculously, all four survived, but if I were to tell their story here, it would fill an entire book, so let me just say that after the war, my older sister, Louise, was six years old, Marianne was four, and they had been shifted back and forth between various safe houses, never quite knowing where they would be the next day. For two years, their lives were but leaves about to fall, and their survival, thanks to courageous Dutchmen, was a true miracle. Yet, I knew nothing of their stories because it had all taken place before I was born.

I am a baby boomer, a child born after the Apocalypse. I came into the tiny island of life in a wasteland of overwhelming death that was our family.

I was born 10 months after the liberation. And even that I did not know. Now that I have knowledge of most of the events that took place before my noisy entrance into their silent world, from documents I uncovered and my personal research, I can share it with anyone willing to listen. Much of my information came from my sisters, but they were so young then, that their memory is necessarily questionable, and much of what they were able to pass on to me came from stories they were told.

My parents never spoke directly to me about the war, so, I had only a few bare facts: they had been in hiding, although I didn't really know why; I had two sisters who each had more than one set of parents, and they had siblings who were not mine. During my early childhood, my sisters disappeared during the summer holidays when they visited their other family. I was jealous of their extended family, and from stories they told me about my early years, I apparently spent a lot of energy trying to collect some extra mamas and papas, brothers, and sisters, so that I could be like them.

So, before I was born, the family had been boisterous and during celebrations their numbers had filled the house to overflowing. That same house where we now sat around a table with room to spare. They had had so much fun together. They had all lived within walking distance, but now all that had been destroyed, and aside from the four portraits of my stern-looking, unsmiling, and unmoving grandparents in black and white along the staircase, an uncle and aunt on the mantle, I did not know there had been so many more whose DNA I shared.

Before I was born, the family had been smiling and loved to tell jokes. By the time I was born, the remnant had fallen silent, and I often thought that perhaps my birth had destroyed their ability to smile, not what had happened before I came into the world.

Knowing what I know today about everything my parents lost, my heart breaks to think I was not more understanding when I was little, but how could I have been, considering no one ever said a word.

Being oblivious to the world that had been stolen from me before I was even born, not being exposed to stories of grandparents and other relatives, except in passing, as if I did not need to hear about them; as if I already knew, my parents gave me a view of my ancestry that was blurred and completely wrong. Perhaps we were a little like Adam and Eve, a first generation, but we certainly did not live in Paradise, the way they had, although we were naked. Naked, vulnerable, and extremely defensive about everything connected to our Jewishness. Although everyone in the village knew we were Jews, it was a secret. It created a world askew, and perhaps that is the best way to describe the world I was given.

We Are Family: A Journey With the 2G Discussion List

Not many Dutch Jews returned from the camps. 104,000 perished there. Of the 36,000 Jews in the post-war Netherlands, perhaps 7,000 had survived the camps. All the others had survived by going into hiding. Arithmetic is not my strong suit, but it is fairly simple: anyone my age was born into a family of survivors, and anyone older than me was actually a Shoah survivor. And yet, no one spoke about those years of occupation and persecution. The survivors shared the same secret and offered their children a topsy-turvy world where madness was the norm. The world I grew up in counted between 30,000 and 40,000 Jews, living among a population of 12 million, more or less. Not even a drop in the sea.

How to explain that world? As an adult graduate student, when I studied Samuel Becket's theatre of the absurd, I understood. That was my world: characters living in garbage cans, waiting for something that would never happen, or speaking doublespeak, yet they made perfect sense to me. Not so much the words, but the ambience, the threat and the horror hanging in the air. I had actually grown up in Samuel Becket's theatre of the absurd, and like his characters, I thought that this was normal. I searched for the same impossible scenes when I played with my friends outside but had a hard time pinpointing what made me feel as if my world was always titled sideways so far that I was about to fall off.

The adults I met when I started Hebrew school, or later, when I joined B'nei Akiva and visited in Amsterdam, Rotterdam, and Hague, all had stories similar to mine, as did their children, who, like me, were also kept in the dark. The mothers were nervous, more jittery than the non-Jewish mothers on my street, and the friends I made sometimes had brothers or sisters much older than them, or there were photos on the mantle of children who had once existed. The older children were foster siblings, Jewish orphans whose parents had not survived.

The husband and wife who ran our Hebrew school had no children. They sometimes spoke of "the child" but he was not there. Instead, they were raising her sister's three children. The young man who maintained my father's typewriter came from a town not too far from us. He, too, was an orphan, nervous and afraid, and always looking over his shoulder. He stammered a little when he spoke. He grew up in his neighbor's home, together with his younger brother and sister. What exactly had happened to his parents was not clear to me either. I constructed stories to explain it all to myself, but never shared any of them with others. When I learned the truth, it was much more horrible than what I had imagined. "The child" my Hebrew teacher mentioned softly to his wife had been entrusted to a farmer who had starved the child to death and pocketed the jewelry he had received in payment. My father's typewriter technician had parents who had made a pact with their neighbors. Whoever survived, would look after the children. One set of parents survived, but their children were lost, so they took in the three orphans and raised them till they were old enough to go out into the world.

The world before I was born was a dark, threatening shadow that hung over everything we did, and sometimes invaded our perfectly appointed, beautifully clean home. It scattered ashes on the carpet that I did not see. I just felt the heat of the grey coal, the icy heat, and tried to ignore it.

Life Before I Knew How to Define Being a 2G

I can unequivocally state that Bnei Akiva first saved and then molded my Jewish identity. This religious Zionist youth movement chose our village as their camping site when I was 9 or 10 years old. A few dozen Jewish youth from Amsterdam and surroundings pitched their tents on the grounds of one of the farms in the village. When the weather was good, they prayed outside. The farmer observed how the person leading the service had wrapped himself in his prayer shawl, the *tallit*, and stopped his chores to observe, then talk to the man. He waited respectfully until the service was over and even kept his cap on, contrary to what he would do in church. "There is someone in the village who had the same priest-robe as you," he told Meier Meier, the owner of the tallit, and the man who had come to the Netherlands to rebuild the youth movement and thus to raise the morale of the child survivors.

The year was 1956 more or less, and all those camping in Nijverdal were indeed children who had lived through the Shoah. Meier Meier was an Israeli educator who had put his career on hold to work as a *shaliah* (emissary) from Israel. Despite his broken Dutch, he immediately understood that the farmer was talking about a Jew who lived in the area. "Does this man still live nearby?" he enquired. Unfortunately, the original owner of the "priest-robe" had long passed away, but the farmer knew that the son or grandson remained in Nijverdal. He gave Meier a name, the men shook hands, and the *shaliah* knew he had to find this Jew whose ancestors had apparently prayed out in the open, just like he and his charges had done now.

That afternoon, someone rang our doorbell. When I opened the door, I found a tall, bronzed man standing outside, looking all exotic and not at all like one of the villagers. I did not understand what he was trying to say, so I ran to call my mother, who came to the door and then ran into the store to call my father, who closed the store and invited the stranger and his companion/translator to come inside. After an emotional exchange of information, my mother served tea and cookies which she assured the men were kosher, and at the end of this amazing meeting, my two older sisters packed a small bag and left with the *shaliah* to join the campers. That Shabbath, my father took my hand and we walked to the campsite. For the first time in my life, I watched my father being called up to the Torah. He knew the blessings without stumbling, tears streaming down his face. I had never seen a Jewish prayer service. Never seen a Torah scroll. Never seen so many Jewish boys and girls.

My sister's counsellor quickly became her fiancé, then husband. I joined Bnei Akiva the next summer when I was 11 years old. I was so impressed by everything there that for days I could not speak. I was also embarrassed of my accent which gave me away as a child from the *Mediene*, but I quickly picked up the swallowed consonants and elongated vowels that typify the speech of Amsterdam, Mokum. That year, I forged friendships that have survived the years. Bnei Akiva nurtured me and sent me on seminars where I learned about the history of the Jews in ancient times, and a little about the more recent history of Shoah. Bnei Akiva eventually offered me a scholarship to study in Israel when I had finished high school and trained me to lead the movement back in the Netherlands. To my shame, however, I did not hold up that end of my bargain as I got married to a nice Jewish American boy whom I had met in Jerusalem and moved to Brooklyn instead.

It would have been so easy to make the transition from country mouse to city mouse and to settle into being a Jewish mama in a city filled with Jewish families, overflowing with Jewish services, kosher food, synagogues, and Jewish day schools, but I was incapable of letting go of that magical year I had lived in Jerusalem, Kevutzat Yavne, and Kibbutz Sde Eliyahu as part of my training. I could not imagine raising children anywhere but in Israel, and my husband was of the same mind. Those children came quickly – within two years we were the parents of two little boys.

The American family I had married into seemed to have no connection to Shoah. Their families had come from Poland and Russia before WWI or shortly after. They were a boisterous, close-knit family, and I loved having so many aunts and uncles. To them I was "the refugee from Europe" and was treated with kindness and a little condescension. It took me a while to pick up the Brooklyn accent, and for the first year I was silent, absorbing sounds and vocabulary. My high school English blossomed and after a while I spoke like my father-in-law, the Brooklyn taxi driver. And yet, America was not my home. For almost five years, to quote the great medieval poet and physician Yehuda Halevi, I was a dweller in the west, in a strange land, learning strange traditions, but my heart was in the east. After nearly five years in America, I was able to answer the call of my heart, and shortly after the Six-Day-War, after my husband had completed his graduate studies, we made *Aliyah* (immigrated to Israel).

My second-generation status, and the fact that my parents and two older sisters were survivors, had all receded into the background. While I understood that the terrible loss of family had left them lonely and perhaps sad, I could not fathom how their years of running for their lives, hiding here, there, and everywhere like prey to the hounds and hunters, had marked them, and how their trauma and the lack of family had also been passed on to me. I compared my parents' status to that of my American family. They had pulled themselves up by their bootstraps, as my mother-in-law liked to say every time someone complained about the difficulties of life. She had no patience for such nonsense. Their life had also been difficult. They were children of immigrants who had struggled with poverty and had achieved what they had achieved with their own two hands. What could I say? Aside from the dead people's portraits that adorned my parents' home, I thought that there was a lot of similarity between the two families. How wrong is wrong? I would soon find out.

I chose to live in Israel because I wanted my children to be surrounded by Jews and I never wanted them to question their identity. I wanted their Jewishness to be as natural as breathing. I wanted them to be free. I also wanted me to be free. Little did I know that my second-generation status had already made that all but impossible. As of yet, I had not heard of any organized groups of people with backgrounds similar to my own. I saw myself as rather unique, considering that our family had been one single Jewish one in a village far from Jewish communities. I did not yet know how enormous the loss of life had been. How sudden and cruel. How final. Eventually, I also learned that my American in-law family had not escaped the Shoah unscathed.

My mother-in-law had had a brother who had left Poland and gone to France when his father and oldest brother left for America. The rest of the family had stayed behind in Poland, to be brought over when there was enough money for tickets, but he decided not to join the rest of the family in America. He got married and had two daughters. And then Hitler came. The entire family was deported to a camp, and he and his daughters were murdered. Only the wife survived.

Years passed. The American side of the family had assumed their brother was gone, and they had never made any attempt to find survivors. The wife eventually located the family in New York, and when the connection remained distant and formal, she eventually wrote them a scathing letter that said that she would never forgive them for not having looked for her and her family after the war. My American family claimed that too much time had passed, and like them, the widow, childless and alone should learn about those bootstraps they had pulled themselves up by.

At the time, I took the entire story at face value. Had not my own parents lived on after the war? I did not know what exhausting efforts my father had made to locate survivors, restore possessions to those few he found, and to claim the inheritance that remained after the murders, and which had been claimed by the Dutch coffers after the war. He spent all his good years on reclaiming everything that had been lost. But I did not know. Perhaps I tried to be like my mother-in-law: pulling on my bootstraps, but I did not quite succeed in staying upright. The bootstraps kept pulling me down, down into the memory of my grandparents and extended family. Down into the experience of my parents who had been forced to relinquish the custody of their young daughters, and to hand them over to the resistance, hoping the children would survive.

In Israel, the commemoration of the six million is a part of the calendar. A day is set aside to mark the Shoah, the murder and heroism of its victims. Everything stops. Television broadcasts deal only with its events, and schools hold ceremonies. Slowly, the realization dawned that I was more part of this than I cared to admit. I asked my big sister who lived in Jerusalem with her survivor husband and their children. She denied any need for commemoration. She wanted only to stand between her children and the memory, and as a result, in her home too, everything was off kilter, the unspoken much louder than the fairy tales of safe haven and normality, just like it had been in my childhood home.

Like my parents, my sister looked at life as if it had begun with her and her husband. Everything that happened before they got married was irrelevant. As she was my mentor, I tried to do the same thing. When I failed to set aside the fact that our grandparents and uncles and aunts had been the victims of that murder machine, she chastised me, saying that all that mattered was Israel and living here, and that all that had happened in Europe was behind us. But it was not. When she was asked to speak at an international conference for hidden children, held in Amsterdam, she refused even to participate. "All of them, wallowing in their past! You will not find me there! The Syrians are threatening the Golan Heights. I must talk about that!" And with those words, she gave me a look never to discuss any of it with her again.

The last time my father visited Israel was shortly after the Yom Kippur War, in the spring of 1974, and while he was here, the son of one of our neighbors, wounded in that war, succumbed to his injuries. My father was devastated, although he knew neither the young man nor his parents. The funeral cortege passed by our house, and he insisted on following the bier. He cried. Parents losing sons. That was too much to bear. I think that that moment I understood something about loss. Yes, his children had survived, but for more than two years he had had no idea of their whereabouts, and when they were returned to him, those years were forever lost. Moreover, he already knew that there no longer was an extended family, grandparents, aunts and uncle, cousins. All gone. Loss that festers through the generations.

I would find out what had happened to my family, but slowly, and I would find out ever more slowly how that loss of people I had never known had left a stamp on me even before I was born. I would find out that there were many people like me living in Israel, America, Europe, Australia, and that we all shared something of that terrible trauma of being the children of survivors of Shoah, and how that created a bond we could not even begin to put into words. What we could do, was understand how we had been touched by this cataclysmic event, and how we could perhaps, perhaps, help each other. I am, of course, talking about the 2G List, which entered my life when I was already the mother of six, grandmother of five, held a tenured job as an English teacher, and was about to start my slow path toward a PhD, while at the same time I was watching how my marriage slowly disintegrated.

Life With the 2G List

I am an observant Jew and I have a strong faith in G-d steering the world, steering my world. I hold with the notion that life is not a matter of chance, but that someone is leading me on my path. The choice to follow the pebbles strewn to show me the way is mine, however, and looking back, I know that I have often taken no heed of those pebbles, and instead have taken circuitous routes that have led me completely astray. Still, that is the premise of free choice, an important precept in Judaism. I believe that as a Jew, I have often taken the road less traveled by, but as I look back, I also know that this has made all the difference. Several compasses have led me.

First and foremost, of course, there was the compass of Jewish observance and the belief that my destiny as a Jew would be to join my brethren in Israel and contribute to building up the ancient homeland. Later on, as

I became more aware of my parents' tragic history, I also tried to follow the road that many children of Shoah survivors must walk, but, as with everything in my life, it took me time to find my fellow Second Generation siblings, so to speak. I had so many aims and objectives, and it has taken me a while to understand that all my obstacles were connected to the fact that I was born shortly after my parents knew for certain that their entire world had been destroyed by the Nazi murder machine, and they were left orphans in a world that was less than welcoming.

I wanted a big family, perhaps to compensate for the silent Jewish holidays of my youth, with my mother setting a festive table, cooking traditional foods and then there were only the six of us. Mother, father, four daughters. No synagogue and no grandparents who came by. The silence was so oppressive that I got away from there as soon as I came of age. I got married young and moved thousands of miles from the village of my birth and childhood.

My weight had been the bane of my existence, and the cause of much friction with my mother, and I truly tried to get my eating disorder under control. Eventually, living in Israel, mother to a large brood, teaching, living in a community I liked very much, I heard about OA, Overeaters Anonymous, and joined a group in my area. It was an eye opener, and I worked the program religiously. Even while on vacation, I made sure there was a meeting somewhere.

While in Jerusalem for a long weekend, I attended an English language meeting for religious women, and met a nice young mother from Beth Shemesh, who stayed after the meeting, so we could talk in private. Among other things, she told me that she was the daughter of survivors. She told me about her family back in the States, and how she and her husband had chosen to raise their large family in Israel. She had recently joined an international email group for children of Shoah survivors who communicated in English. The idea of such an organization intrigued me. As of yet, I had no idea that in spite of our differences, we shared so much based on our parents' experiences during WWII.

I joined The List. Until that moment I had genuinely believed that most of my quirky behaviors, my sense of isolation and of being different from the rest of the world were the result of having grown up in a small village on the German border as the one Jewish family there. I had given no real thought to everything that had been taken from my parents – and thus from us, their children as well – by a cruel and horrible pogrom that lasted 5 years and murdered 75 out of every 100 Dutch Jews, leaving a devastated remnant with little or no infrastructure to live their lives as Jews.

At first, I shared very little of my background. I felt shy. I wanted to see what people were saying to each other, but when I was asked to write a short bio about my background, questions started, and they made me think. Every day, I got up a little earlier to read the messages from The List, and I was shocked to realize that so many of the members grappled with similar issues. Many had had painful and difficult relationships with their parents. Many had not known what had happened to their parents. Some had had siblings they never knew, yet whose portraits hung above their beds. Many grew up in homes of perpetual mourning.

The List became my second home. It helped me to understand something about my marriage. I was not happy and had long felt tied down in a relationship that had stagnated, but I could not leave. I owed it to my husband to stay. I did not realize that I was entitled to feel different about myself. Not everything could be discussed over the public List, but I forged strong friendships with 2G members who allowed me to write privately, off-List. I opened up everything. To people I had never met. To people I thought I might never even meet. They lived in Canada, Australia, America. I was in Israel, and not a very frequent traveler.

Many of my 2G friends were divorced. Many were over-achievers, but some were happy in long-surviving unions, and some were not college graduates. We all shared intense relationships with our children, whether good and nurturing or angry and distant. The feelings were larger than life. I found that my fellow 2Gs lived like me, in capital letters, feeling everything just a little more strongly than those not on that List, and that almost all of us were struggling with issues of identity and belonging.

The List accepted me for who I was and was not afraid to call me to task when they felt I was doing life all wrong. We were siblings on some level, and we were allowed to tell each other what we were thinking. We had shouting matches over the email List, and some of us left in a huff, or were unlisted because they could not accept the framework of listening and responding. I loved that List. I loved that List, and I am grateful to all who joined and passed through. I loved the people I shared so much with, and eventually, I got to meet quite a few of them. We grew into an international community, bound by common experience, and protective of each other. I was never afraid that anyone of The List would betray my confidences.

Of course, more of its members traveled to Israel than the other way around. When a group member came, the Israeli contingent got busy, and organized a get-together. Almost all of us showed up, happy and smiling. Some silent, and some noisy. Some for the entire meeting, others just to say hello. But we showed up.

My Australian friend and her husband were globe-trotters, and they asked if I would come to Italy to meet them. I agreed – an impulsive notion, but there I was. We would spend a weekend in Florence, and I was put in charge of organizing kosher food. The first lap of my journey left me in Pisa, and the plan was to meet there in the morning and tour the city. I had barely put down my suitcase in an amazing hotel that used to be a convent, when I got a message to come to the lobby. My Aussie friends had decided they could not wait another day and had taken the train to surprise me. We were like long-lost relatives. It was liberating and amazing, and we spent an absolutely magical weekend together. They walked to the ancient synagogue with me, and we had no food because the hotel had no fridge, and everything spoiled. But never mind! We had each other. Of course, I missed my flight home and did not make it back to the classroom on time. I made some excuse about a sick sister, and all was forgiven.

Just before earning my PhD in literature, I was invited to Boston for the international ALA conference, to give a paper entitled "A Jewish Reading of Arthur Miller's *All My Sons*", and after the conference I was set to meet one of our 2G members who would take me on a tour of the city. We discovered that we could sit and talk for hours, and again, the connection was immediate and simple. At the end of an exhausting day of sight-seeing, they dropped me off at the airport and I flew to Canada to spend time with another member of The List. There, too, the connection was instantaneous, and we hugged like we had been searching for each other for years. Well, perhaps there was some truth in that...

Visits were reciprocal. Quite a few members couch-surfed and spent time with each other. Once, I hosted a weekend for people from Israel and abroad, and my house filled up with middle-aged plus women who acted like teenagers.

The List has been through many ups and downs. At times it has been silent. At times it has been crackling with activity. During the year of Corona, we managed to have virtual meetings through Zoom. It was all wonderful. Every time I get a message with the name of one of my 2G friends – be it on The List, on Facebook or any other way – I am happy. Those are my friends. I know I am welcome at their home, and they are welcome in mine. I have attended the circumcision ceremony of the child of at least one of our members and met other 2Gs who happened to be in Israel and had made the effort to attend as well. I have mourned the passing of people I never met in person, but who were important to one of the members of The List, and I have tried to comfort them. I have attended the zoom-funeral of one of us and remembered what a lovely time we had together when she came to Israel.

I believe that being on The List has honed my identity. But more than that: I have made my peace with my 2G status. I no longer need to kick and scream at the world about this. Being a child of survivors has helped me to clarify who I am. In a way it has contributed to my professional identity and area of interest and research, and in a way, it has influenced the way I communicate with my children and grandchildren. Perhaps being a child of survivors is a badge of honor, for it proves unequivocally that our parents chose life. We are the living proof that the Jewish People Live – *AM YISRAEL HAY* – and for this I am grateful.

Notes on Contributors

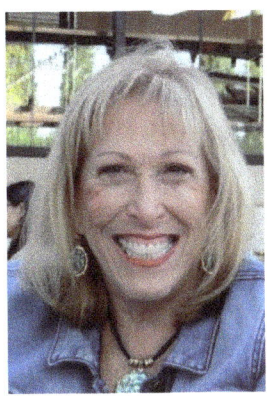

Marilyn Boehm was born in Kingston, New York in 1949 after traveling by U.S. naval ship from a German Displaced Persons camp with her Hungarian Holocaust survivor parents and three-year-old sister. As her parents "golden child", she took ballet lessons, joined the Girl Scouts, and engaged in many traditionally American activities to make her parents proud. She was editor of her junior high and high school newspapers and went on to achieve a Magna Cum Laude B.A. degree from Cal State University at Northridge. She retired in 2004 after 31 years of service as a deputy probation officer. Since then, she has been an avid world traveler, exploring other cultures and religious beliefs. She calls Huntington Beach, California home, where she lives with her husband and two adorable dogs. Her passion for animals has led to involvement as a district leader of the US Humane Society. She also cherishes visits with her two adult children and three grandchildren. She is the published author of the memoir *Starting at Goodbye*.

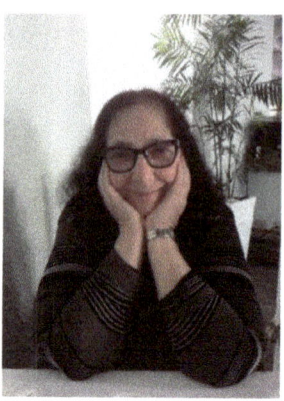

Dr. Paula David is the proud mother of five very adult children and four of the best grandchildren ever. Together with her husband Lee, she is happiest when surrounded by family and friends. Paula is a partially retired professor, lecturing part time in Gerontology at the University of Toronto and Ryerson University. Since her official "retirement" she still does part time lecturing, consulting, and studying in her field, these days, from a very personal perspective. As an older woman facing age related rewards and challenges, she continues to seek new friendships, adventures, and insights. She thoroughly enjoys tea parties and just hanging out with her grandkids, plays her flute in a klezmer band, maintains her community volunteer work, and has rediscovered the joys of drawing and painting. Inspired by her years as a member of the 2ndGen Listserv, she is currently collecting and writing the inherited narratives and tales of her ancestors.

Notes on Contributors

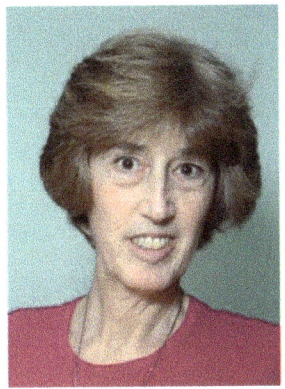

Patrice Flesch was born in Manhattan and was raised in the suburb of Garden City, Long Island. She received a B.S. in Communications. After five years of working at jobs she disliked, she returned to school to study photography. From there, she went on to become a free-lance photographer and had an exciting career meeting famous people and going to places that she otherwise wouldn't have been able to. With her career in place, she married her beloved husband Peter Rogers. Eventually, she turned to teach her lifelong study of yoga at her award-winning studio and was a pioneer in teaching yoga to people who have Alzheimer's. Simultaneously, she worked for the New England Holocaust Memorial as a docent. Due to illness, both she and her husband retired early. Patrice then became almost a full-time volunteer as an advocate for people living in poverty. Because she wanted to spend the bulk of her time living in Mexico, she founded her own online organization Action Against Anti-Semitism. Due to her personal experiences, she wants to spend her remaining years fighting antisemitism.

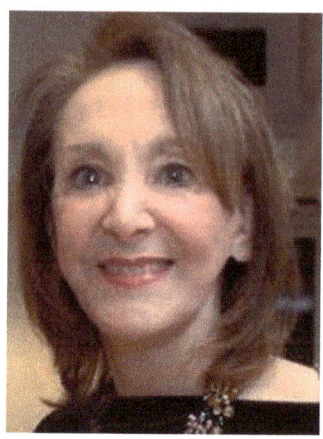

Dr. Eva Fogelman is a social psychologist, psychotherapist, author, and filmmaker. She is in private practice in New York City and was co-founder and co-director of Psychotherapy with Generations of the Holocaust and Related Traumas at Training Institute for Mental Health, and Jewish Foundation for Christian Rescuers, ADL (Jewish Foundation for the Righteous), currently co-director Child Development Research (includes International Study of Organized Persecution of Children). Dr. Fogelman is co-editor of several books on the psychological and historical perspective on children during the Nazi reign and its aftermath. She is the writer and co-producer of the award-winning documentary *Breaking the Silence: The Generation After the Holocaust* (PBS). Dr. Fogelman is a Pulitzer Prize nominee for *Conscience and Courage: Rescuers of Jews During the Holocaust*. Her hundreds of writings appear in professional as well as popular publications. Dr. Fogelman is a pioneer in therapeutic interventions for generations of the Holocaust and related historical traumas and is a frequent consultant and speaker nationally and internationally.

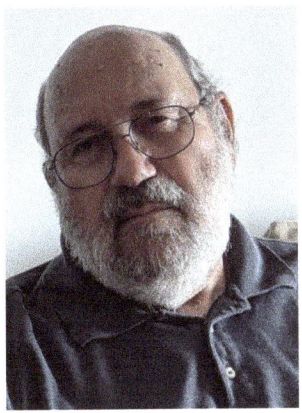

Paul Foldes is a first-generation immigrant from Hungary. After arriving in the USA, he grew up in New York City, where he attended public schools, including the highly competitive merit-based Stuyvesant High School. He is a graduate of New York University's School of Engineering (BE, Electrical Engineering) and Georgetown University's Law Center (JD) His career started as a consumer protection attorney at the Federal Trade Commission where he was co-counsel on several landmark cases and rulemaking that continue to significantly benefit consumers to the present. After leaving the FTC he became a successful business and social impact entrepreneur. He considers his son to be his greatest success, and his grandchildren to be his teachers of early childhood experiences and lessons, something that he missed out on as a child of Holocaust survivors in Communist Hungary.

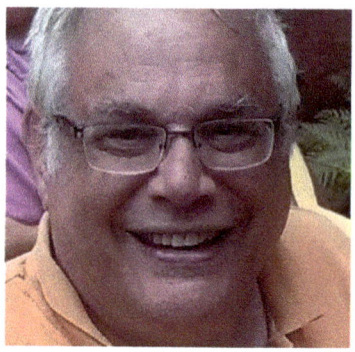

Martin Herskovitz was born in the United States in 1955 to parents from Czechoslovakia, his mother a Holocaust survivor. He completed a BA in psychology at Yeshiva University and an MA in safety and occupational hygiene at NYU. In 1986, Martin, his wife, Pearl, and two sons, immigrated to Israel where their daughter was born. After a position as a work supervisor at the Ministry of Labor, 1989 Martin began his work as a safety officer at the logistic center in the IDF, a role he fulfilled until his retirement in 2018. Martin began a Second-generation activity in 2000 as part of a listserv of the Second Generation, in which he began to publish poetry in the field of Second Generation experiences. His poems were published in *Midstream* and *Maggid*. On the basis of his poems, he prepared a lecture on the subject of "Poetry and Second generation" which he presented at the University of Illinois, Leslie University in Israel and twice at the annual educators' conference at Yad Vashem. After retiring from the IDF, Martin began to increase his activities in the field of Holocaust remembrance, became a Public Fellow at the Finkler Institute of Holocaust Research at Bar-Ilan University, and founded the "Creating Memory", an arts-based program, to insure the continuation of the narrative in future generations.

Notes on Contributors

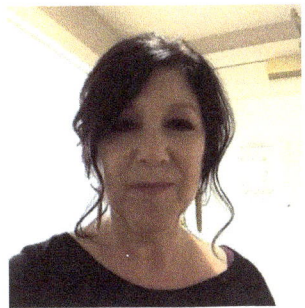

Clara Jacob grew up in St. Paul, Minnesota, USA. She received a BA in English from Vassar College and an MFA in Creative Writing from Goddard College. Clara has worked in advertising and marketing for many years, has taught college-level English and writing, and co-wrote a book with her daughter, *Our Sisters' Voices: Teenage Girls of Color Speak Out*. She currently lives in South Dakota. Clara has three adult children and three grandchildren.

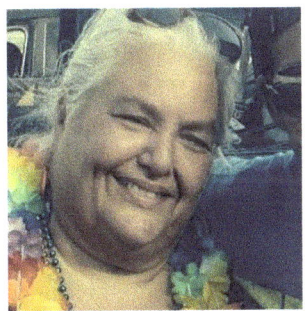

Gail Ellen Rubinstein Lipton, a child of the fifties, grew up on Long Island. After completing her B.S. and M.S. Ed. degrees from the University of Pennsylvania, she remained in Philadelphia, where she met her husband, Barry. Through the years Gail has taught in both public and private schools, has been both a religious-school teacher and principal, and also established a synagogue Talmud Torah. She has been a federal employee since the late 1970s and is currently employed within the Health Resources and Services Administration, an agency within the Department of Health and Human Services, where she serves as a Senior Advisor and subject matter expert on financial assistance, health workforce policy development, and related management information system and training issues. She has received numerous job-related honors and awards, including the Secretary's Award for Distinguished Service and the Administrator's Citation for Outstanding Performance. An empty nester, Gail currently resides in Maryland with her husband. When not working she enjoys reading, music, and going to concerts.

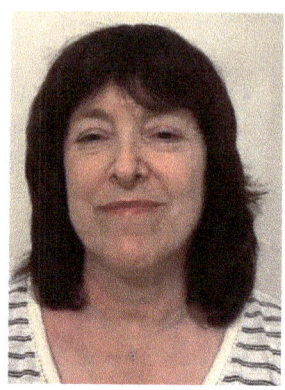

Dr. Betty Unger Needleman's life began in Brooklyn, New York, in a close-knit family encompassing doting and protective parents, and an older brother. Both of her parents were Holocaust survivors from a small town in southeast Poland. They both lost countless loved ones during the war years, senselessly murdered at the hands of the Nazis. When her parents were at home, their primary language was Yiddish; however, when they did not want their children to understand, they spoke Polish. Betty attended university in Buffalo, NY, and afterwards attended graduate school in Ohio. After getting married, she and her husband lived in Philadelphia, PA for several years while he attended school, and even after his graduation. Eventually, they decided to relocate back towards home. As a result of the Holocaust, Betty did not have the opportunity to know her grandparents. Her husband, on the other hand, knew all his grandparents and enjoyed a loving relationship with them. Therefore, they wanted their future children to know and love their parents. As a result, they reside in central New Jersey, where they raised our own family. They continue to work, and fortunately now enjoy the special "club" of being grandparents. Becoming a parent and now grandparent is the biggest, most meaningful, and important privilege of Betty's life.

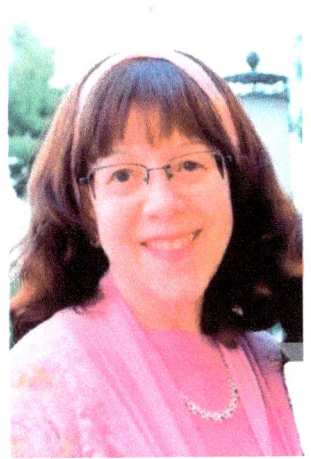

Prof. Judith Tydor Baumel-Schwartz was born in New York in 1959 and immigrated to Israel with her Holocaust survivor father and American-born mother in 1974. She completed her undergraduate and graduate degrees at Bar-Ilan University and specializes in Holocaust Studies and Israel Studies with emphasis on gender, memory, and religion. She has written and edited numerous books and articles about religious life during and after the Holocaust, gender and the Holocaust, Holocaust commemoration, public memory in the State of Israel, and studies about descendants of Holocaust survivors. Today she directs the Arnold and Leona Finkler Institute of Holocaust Research at Bar-Ilan University where she is a Professor of Modern Jewish History. She is married to Prof. Joshua Schwartz and together they have a blended family of children and grandchildren.

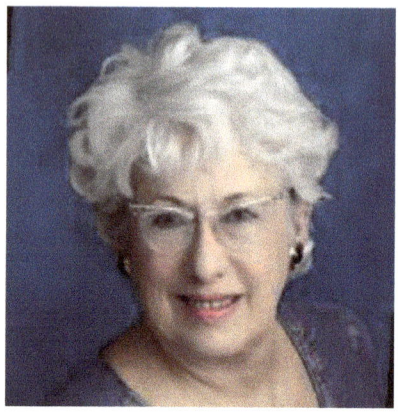

Jeanette Friedman Sieradski, born in Bed-Stuy and basically raised in Haredi Brooklyn, is a lover of Yiddish theater, author, journalist, editor, activist, mother, grandma, and great-grandma on a different *derech* (path). She now lives in a log cabin in the Pocono Mountains. After almost 50 years as a leader in Second Generation, a lay educator and publisher of Holocaust memoirs at The Wordsmithy, she trains students to interview Holocaust survivors for Names Not Numbers. She is currently working on the establishment of a Holocaust and Genocide Study and Resource Center in Monroe County, PA. Most importantly, she's "gotta have House Music, all night long" to keep the blood pumping and the spirit up.

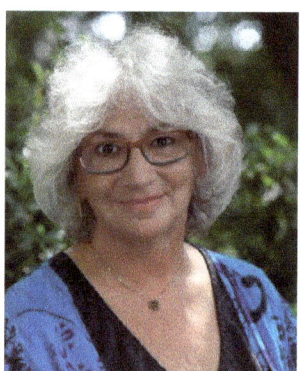

Laurie Solnik is a longtime resident of Washington, DC. After retiring from her Federal career as a Government Relations Representative for the US Postal Service, Laurie became the full-time lay leader of Hill Havurah, a vibrant, independent Jewish community on Capitol Hill which she helped found. Laurie holds degrees from Boston University and the New York Institute of Technology. She remains active in progressive causes, rescues stray animals and humans, tutors B'nai Mitzvah students and dotes on her grandchildren.

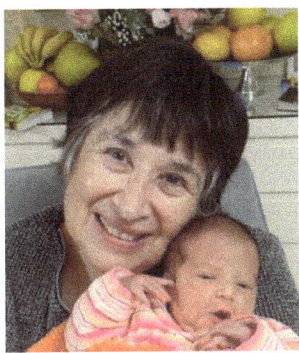

Dr. Ruth Samuel Tenenholtz was born in a small village in the Netherlands, in 1946, the third daughter in a family of Holocaust survivors. Her parents were virtually the only survivors of their large, extended family. Despite the Holocaust they remained Orthodox Jews, and she grew up with a strong Jewish identity, while knowing little about what had taken place before she was born. Marrying young, she lived in America for nearly five years, and immigrated to Israel with her husband and two young sons in 1969. Having completed her education in Israel, eventually earning a PhD in English literature, she also gave birth to four more children. Today, after many years as a lecturer in various frameworks, she is retired and writes books and articles which deal with the Holocaust in the Netherlands. Seventy-five years after the catastrophe that decimated the Jewish people, she feels that something has been repaired for her large family. They are once again a tribe with parents, children, grandchildren, and great-grandchildren, all of whom she enjoys. Best of all, in her opinion, is the fact that they are living, working, and raising children in Israel, the Jewish homeland.

www.ingramcontent.com/pod-product-compliance
Ingram Content Group UK Ltd.
Pitfield, Milton Keynes, MK11 3LW, UK
UKHW021256180426
11947UKWH00011B/811